Mesmerism Practicum

The Secret Art Of Mesmerism

A Vademacum of the divine techniques of Mesmerism, Fascination and Non-Verbal Hypnosis that may be used to aide and help our fellow man. The first part being comprised of the techniques and exercises needed to learn this art, the second parts dedicated to using it to help physically and emotionally heal yourself and others and the third dedicated to the more curious forms of the art including clairvoyance and long distance healing.

Jason Healy

Copyright © 2024 by Jason Healy

All rights reserved.

No portion of this book may be reproduced in any form without written permission from the publisher or author, except as permitted by U.S. copyright law. This publication is designed to provide accurate and authoritative information in regard to the subject matter covered. It is sold with the understanding that neither the author nor the publisher is engaged in rendering legal, investment, accounting or other professional services. While the publisher and author have used their best efforts in preparing this book, they make no representations or warranties with respect to the accuracy or completeness of the contents of this book and specifically disclaim any implied warranties of merchantability or fitness for a particular purpose. No warranty may be created or extended by sales representatives or written sales materials. The advice and strategies contained herein may not be suitable for your situation. You should consult with a professional when appropriate. Neither the publisher nor the author shall be liable for any loss of profit or any other commercial damages, including but not limited to special, incidental, consequential, personal, or other damages.

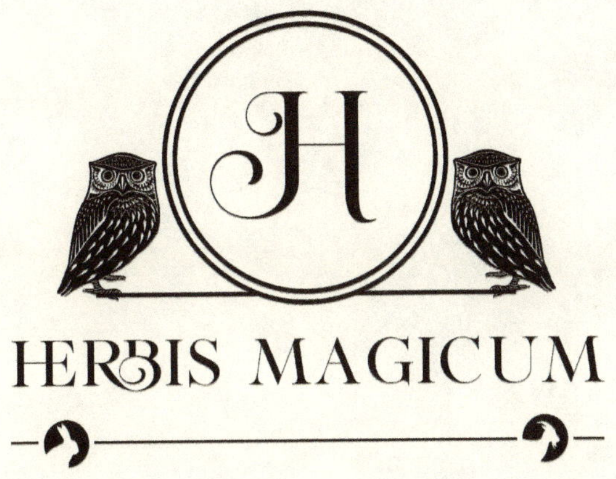

Table Of Contents

Disclaimer:

Information offered in this book is for educational purposes only. We make neither medical claims, nor intend to diagnose or treat medical conditions. Individuals who are pregnant or nursing, and persons with known medical conditions, should consult their licensed health care provider before using any of the techniques in this book. Readers must do their own research concerning the safety and usage of these techniques.

INTRO

Reader you hold in your hands the beginning of the understanding of the divine, the beginning of being able to truly help those around you. Guard this book, study it, and learn the secrets of nature. For those that study these pages will learn the secrets to help heal themselves and those around them. Remember that we do not heal, that is something only the body can do, but we can help it. They say man is a body with a soul but the truth is so much more, for in reality man is a soul with a body. Man's true essence is pure energy, he is part of the divine, and the All lies within him.

We have all heard of auras, and energy fields. These fields are real and are produced by the human body. They are measurable and have been seen. They flow from the top of the head outward around the bottom and down to the floor. They extend away from and around the body. In addition these energy channels run throughout the body. In fact the heart produces one of the strongest energy fields in the body and is up to 2 meters wide around the body. All living things produce this energy, and when we have a blockage or disruption of the energy it can lead to pain and disease, and so by learning to direct the energy and remove the blockages, we can help heal pain and disease in all things from people to animals and even plants.

There are 2 main ways to correct this energy. The first is with herbs as we have discussed in our other work Herbis Magicum. Herbs work both on the physical level but also on the spiritual level, the second is by directing the body's energy. There are several ways to do this including Mesmerism for the west and Qi-gong for the east are the most commonly known. In this book, we will go into the long forgotten depths of Mesmerism and Fascination. I believe to truly heal you must be able to use both energy and herbs, both the physical and the spiritual. And when you are ready, I would suggest you also read our other book Herbis Magicum as this will give you an excellent beginning in herbs and how to use them in a spiritual sense before taking them into a higher level with alchemy.

Mesmerism works on 2 main principles. The first is on non-verbal hypnosis which is far more effective than verbal hypnosis. Because in verbal hypnosis even though the person is under a hypnotic influence they still must stay somewhat conscious to hear and understand the verbal commands. With non-verbal hypnosis people go much deeper and much faster due to not having to keep the conscious mind engaged. In addition, while verbal hypnosis does not work on everyone, non verbal hypnosis does. And so you have a much higher success rate with it, and you are not limited to language patterns, in fact it doesn't even matter if the person speaks the same language as you or not. In addition because the person is in a deeper state of hypnosis it allows the brain to change brainwaves and thus enter a much deeper healing state. Oftentimes a person will be healed after one session of Mesmerism, where they had not been healed before after many conventional tries.

The second principle that Mesmerism works on, is the movement of blocked energy. It allows us to direct the body's energy of the person or thing that needs it. It is always with us, everywhere, and we may call on it in a moment's notice, when we have nothing else, because it already lies within us. This energy, this essence, is intelligent and knows what is needed from it. It goes where it is needed, heals what is sick, and balances that which is out of balance. It is said to be the essence, the ether, but I believe it is the All, that lies within us and surrounds us. The very essence of God, and thus Mesmerism is sacred, it is a gift of healing, and its knowledge brings us just a little closer to the All, and so it must be always respected.

For within this sacred knowledge lies the ability to help heal those who suffer. Today, sadly we view the body as mechanical, if this is wrong you simply correct it with that, if this part breaks you swap it with that. In today's world we swap out organs like a mechanic swaps out engine parts. But the body is not mechanical, it is divine, and all of this is just on the physical level and while this often relieves the issue for a time being another issue shortly pops up. It is because the body is not just physical it is energy and when this energy is disrupted, or blocked we can manifest disease or pain, we say it is because of a germ or infection and while this is what is the cause, the source is due to the energy.

Know that all infirmities, all pains, physical or mental are at the root caused by a disruption in the energy field of man. Remove this blockage and you remove the source of the infirmity. This is true for all living beings. This was the concept Paracelsus once said all those years ago. He also said the only true purpose of magick was to heal. And with this in mind let us begin to learn Magick. This book is designed to take you step by step so you may learn to guide this energy, this essence, this mesmeric fluid and to heal. It is filled with techniques from helping to heal pain, disease, and psychological issues to eliminating phobias, creating clairvoyance, and seeing things in magic mirrors.

Mesmerism is the beginning of very powerful techniques. But remember that it is not the mesmerist that heals a person. So we can never say we healed anyone. All a mesmerist is, is an empty vessel for this energy to flow into a person. But it is always the person that heals themselves. All Mesmerism does is aids the body to heal naturally. What is in this book can not be used to harm, so that you can do no wrong with it. Which is great, you don't have to worry about too much or too little, or doing something wrong, as the energy is intelligent and knows what is needed of it.

It's history is long and fascinating. It was Franz Anton Mesmer who is credited with discovering it. Using these techniques he reportedly helped so many people in Paris that the medical establishment got scared and kicked him out of France, declaring him a fraud, because he was supposedly helping people they could not. Later ofcourse he returned to Paris. One of his most famous followers was the Marquis of Puységur who wrote a book himself and I would suggest you look into it. However while Mesmer is credited with discovering it mesmerism and fascination is a type of ancient Divine knowledge that has been around for centuries and guarded closely.

Mesmerism's past uses are fascinating. In the past it could be used to create energetic barriers that man and animals could not cross, influence the minds of enemies to turn against each other, and even create visions by telepathic thought transference that a person would experience as real. Because it's, energy

It can be used to help heal at great distances. Sounds could be used to entrance, and heal, as well as grow crops.

With the combination of secret symbols drawn on the ground with mesmeric intention, there are stories of it being used to restore a person's very life force, and finally it could be used to glimpse the future and view far off distant places. Most of this knowledge unfortunately has been lost or hidden and it is my hope that by writing this book we may preserve its healing abilities and thus elevate mankind just a little above the diseases he is told he must suffer from. I only share this with you to show you that when I say what you are about to learn is a gift of the divine you will know that I am not just saying poetic words but speaking of a very real truth.

But know that this book is only the beginning. There is so much more a master of mesmerism can do. I encourage the true seeker of knowledge to explore the books of the past and find the techniques not listed here to truly unlock the secrets of mesmerism. However the techniques in this book are all you should need to be able to heal those around you, ...and be able to do a little more. However, this book is useless if you do not study its lessons and practice its exercises. If you have found this book it is for a reason, guard it well.

The book has been designed as a reference book of techniques to be called upon when needed. The first part of each section of the book will teach you the exercises necessary to strengthen your abilities to be able to do the techniques, the second part will teach the techniques, then later it will show you which techniques are needed to help different ailments. In the advanced section we will talk about long distance healing and a few tricks you can do such as creating clairvoyance. Take the book in stages, because knowing the knowledge is useless if you can not do the techniques. It does not take long to learn, dedicate the time needed, and you will find you will become an incredible healer in a very short time.

There are 4 stages of Mesmerism, the 1st stage is fascination, 2nd stage is catalepsy, 3rd stage is somnambulism, and 4th is lethargy. We will talk about these stages throughout the book but for now just know that If you follow these stages in order, you will create stronger trances. You can skip steps, but if you follow the path each step will be stronger by following the last step rather than skipping over it. Because each leads to the next. Fascination begins the process of catalepsy, and many times when you see the person's eyes open during fascination it is because they are already in a small state of catalepsy before you go into a deeper state of it.

(Chapter 1) Fascination

We will start this book with fascination because when a person is fascinated they immediately feel energy. This allows us to magnetize faster and deeper than we normally could without fascination.

Fascination is the ability to look in a person's eyes and entrance them without words. It has a romance about it, to be able to say look into my eyes and have a person succumb to you, to be entranced and seduced by your very will. This one skill will allow you to influence, seduce, entrance, and heal those around you, and is the first skill we will study in this book because it can be used alone, or to increase the strength and speed of magnetism. This is because our eyes are one of the areas that emit this mesmeric energy, this essence, and because of this they can be directed to heal and entrance. All people have this ability, but few know or develop it, but every now and then we come across someone. Have you ever looked into a person's eyes and felt something... almost overpowering?

We see this all the time in the animal world and there are many stories of snakes using this technique to actually draw prey right into their waiting mouths. There was even a story of a man who came across a rattlesnake in his garden. He made the mistake of looking into its eyes and became fascinated and began to call for help that he was going to fall into the snake but there was nothing he could do. Luckily the man's wife threw a rock at the snake which broke the spell and the snake slithered off.

Healing power has always been connected to fascination, and even Hippocrates and Paracelsus both mentioned that healing could be caused by the gaze. It can be used to heal pain and other issues, as well as hypnotize. Fascination allows us to bring the subject into a very primitive mind which is open to our will and to magnetism. And thus its knowledge not only allows us to heal but also influence.

After we put someone in a fascinated state all energetic techniques work better as the subject is more receptive to the energetic technique, and the flow of energy, and because of this, while it's not necessary, it's always better to start a mesmeric treatment with fascination, because not only will the treatment be more effective, but once in a fascinated state you will be able to mesmerize them much faster. In addition once in a fascinated state we can do several things,

1). We can give the subconscious mind commands both non-verbal and verbal, which act like all the different techniques of hypnosis, but more powerfully, as less people can resist it than conventional hypnosis. Bear in mind we can not compel them to do something they would not ordinarily do, like commit a crime or something like that, because their subconscious mind will still protect them. And even if we could do that, we shouldn't, our highest aim should be to help and heal. In addition, often with fascination they won't remember what happened and don't even close their eyes. This loss of memory can happen from deeper states of mesmerism as well. But we will cover those areas later. Once they are fascinated, as an example, we can actually speak directly to the subconscious. You can say "unconscious mind" push the person forward, or push them backward and you will see them move in the direction you tell them. We use the word unconscious, instead of subconscious because we are doing 2 things , first we are addressing the subconscious and it knows this, but by saying unconscious we are also telling it to keep the person unconscious. You could also say something like I am speaking to "Johns unconscious mind" etc. There are also ton of things you can do here that are similar to the push technique, such as making people forget their names, telling them 1+2=4 etc.

2). Another very valuable technique you can do is Anesthesia and Catalepsy. Anethesia is where we can remove pain, and even prevent the person from feeling pain before a treatment like during childbirth or dentistry, or a surgery. We can also achieve

Catalepsy, which is where the person is put in a statue-like state, normally catalepsy and anesthesia go hand in hand so when you see catalepsy, you can be fairly confident they cant feel pain, but it's always good to test. This can be done just with fascination, but can also be done with mesmerism as well, and we will talk about these techniques in more detail in the mesmeric chapters.

3). We can even do a regression with fascination as well. Similar to a hypnotic regression however you can get the person in a regression in seconds rather than the longer times conventional verbal hypnosis needs. Regression is where we can take a person back in time to relive a situation to help them get over a trauma.

So as you can see this is a very useful technique to know for healing, hypnosis, and it also greatly increases our ability to influence in normal conversation as well. The techniques below will begin your journey and teach you all you need to begin to heal, and entrance, but you should also know that just like mesmerism, Fascination, can do much more, again, you will need to look deep in the past to unlock all of its secrets…. if they can be found. But that is half the fun isn't it? In the meantime master what is in this book, and you will have all you need.

Fascination Eye Exercises

To be able to do fascination you must be able to keep your eyes open for up to 15 minutes without blinking. The following exercises will not only increase the power of your gaze but will also increase the power of your influence as well. When you do these exercises you won't be able to do for more than about 30 seconds initially, but as you continue to practice you will see the time increases and eventually you will be able to do it for 5, 10, 15 minutes without blinking. You must feel calm while you do this as this will help you keep your eyes open longer, as when you stare off into space when you are tired. Do not over do these exercises, once you blink stop and you may try them one more time, but that is all for the day. This is the same as the gym you must build up slowly.

1). Tiny Black Dot Exercise

Find a small black point an arm's length away from you, or you can simply draw a small dot on a white piece of paper and place it at arms length away, and stare at it without blinking for as long as you can. Once you blink the exercise is over. You may do it once more if you wish but do not over do it. These techniques take time, but not too much.

2). Reflected Dot Exercise

This is exactly the same as the black dot but it is done by finding a small point with reflected light. Such as a small pinhole where the sunlight hits. It can also be artificial light if necessary. Reflected light affects the brain differently, and so it must be practiced along with the black dot exercise. But the procedure is exactly the same.

3). Mirror Exercise (very important)

It is Very important to develop Magnetic Gaze. As you practice with a mirror, you will get better and better. All the exercises you practice will be stronger with the Mirror. It will also help you transmit to your client what you want, because you have done it yourself with the mirror so it will be easier for your client to feel what you want and do it as well.

Look at the mirror and at your third eye and stare at yourself without blinking. You must be about 20cm away from the mirror. You can set a timer and initially as mentioned you will not be able to do it for more than about 30 seconds as this is the longest a normal person can go without blinking, but as you progress you will notice that you will quickly increase the amount of time before you need to blink. It is important to feel calm in your mind as this will help increase your time before you need to blink. It's similar to when you are tired and stare off into nothingness, you don't need to blink as often. So by feeling calm it puts you in a similar state and will increase your time.

When gazing into the mirror you will begin to go into trance yourself. This can be used to your advantage. As you stare into your third eye in the mirror you will notice your eyes go hazy and you vision changes. This happens because you begin to fascinate yourself and this is how you can begin to do self-hypnosis, as well as self healing. In this state you can also give yourself positive affirmations and program your mind for different successes.

However, when you are using Fascination on someone else, the last thing you want to do is go into trance yourself. To stop this we need something called Presence which we will talk about in a minute. The important thing to know here is that If you are not trying to self hypnotize, when you start to feel your eyes go hazy and everything begins to disappear you can feel presence and you will notice your vision and sensation pops right back in. This is how you can practice to ensure you are not fascinated yourself when you are trying to fascinate someone else.

Note: Alternate 1 day black spot, 1 day reflected spot, and looking at the mirror every day.

Also, In daily life try to do everything you can without blinking. These three exercises are the primary exercises you need to do to get up to speed. The exercises below will augment and improve your ability. But these three should be your primary exercises.

To Increase The Speed Of Your Gaze

Hold your finger up about a foot or 2 from our face then practice looking in the distance and then looking at your finger and alternating your vision back and forth this will increase the speed of your gaze.

Eye Mobility

Hold your 2 hands in thumbs up positions, one on the left side one on the right side and look at the one then the other then look up and down and just alternate between the thumbs moving your eyes and not so much your head. Do this many times.

Sideways 8 Eye Exercise

Look at the mirror and choose a point right in front of you, and then move your head in an infinity design while continuing to always look forward at this point. This increases eye movement, and can also help any lazy eye issues.

Piercing Black Arrows Exercise

Find a point and imagine small black arrows shooting from your eyes towards the point, this will increase the strength of your gaze.

Presence

In all forms of Mesmerism and fascination we must be in presence. In presence, our abilities are stronger and work faster and it prevents us from going into trance ourselves. We are always in our minds thinking constantly, about the future and the past about everything except where we are right here and now. In order to keep yourself from going into trance and being fascinated yourself, you must stop this and be in the present, in the here and now, without thought. This will not only keep you from becoming a victim of your own abilities but quickly decrease the amount of time it takes to put someone else into trance, and heal them, as well as cause them to go much deeper. Presence is of the utmost importance in both fascination and mesmerism so it is a skill you must learn. Luckily it's fairly easy.

And while there are tons of meditations that say to clear your mind the truth is it is almost impossible to stop your thoughts, however there is a trick which will help give you what you need.

Using Presence:

While you are gazing into the mirror, or the person, or even using mesmeric passes which we will talk about later, to be in presence:

1). Feel the sensation of your left hand, you can feel its weight, its heat, feel it attached to your wrist.

2). While feeling the presence of your left hand you also want to feel the gravity holding your feet to the floor, feel your feet and the weight of your body pressing into the floor.

3). While feeling the sensation of your left hand and the gravity holding your feet into the ground, Feel how straight you are standing.

By feeling all these at the same time you will notice your thoughts stop and you are in the here and now. When you are looking in the mirror and start to see the haze and feel yourself going into trance simply go into presence and you will feel yourself pop back.

As I mentioned before, Presence is vital for mesmerism and fascination it must be mastered. It will keep you from going into trance and also allow you to get your subject much deeper much faster so always use presence when you are working with the techniques in this book.

To Practice Presence:

Go around for a few days and every chance you get, keep the 3 sensations in mind and try to stay present as long as you can. You will not be able to do it forever or even for a few hours but your time will build up and if you can use it during normal conversations people will feel you are listening closer to them, it will improve your influence as well as your memory, and your day will seem longer. Which is particularly useful for your weekends.

2nd Exercise To Work On Presence:

Count your breathing, so as you inhale that is 1 as you exhale that is 2 as you inhale that is 3 exhale 4 and you continue until 6 then you start over. This stops the mind and makes you more present.

The Energetic Field

This is where you link with your client. There is a point in the process where you feel your client, as if connected. You are just there without thought. The best way to do this is with presence. But once you have a sensation creating a field of coherence will allow you to entrance much faster and deeper. To get a field of coherence do not visualize and just feel a sensation or emotion, for example calm or peace. To do this we can enter a present state, and then remember a memory that is tied to an emotional state that made you feel this emotion, then recreate this feeling from the memory. Once you feel this calm emotion you can then begin to fascinate or magnetize and you will find you are far more effective, because their mind is able to feel this calm from you as well.

Remember: The subject always feels the emotional state of the practitioner, so stay calm and present.

Using Your Stronger Gaze To Influence In Normal Conversation

Even without putting a person into fascination we can use some techniques to greatly improve our influence, but we have to be careful and not look like serial killers as well. You can begin by looking at people when you talk, but don't stare, just look at them, like a normal person would do without blinking and see what happens. It will also increase your influence. You can even begin to increase your influence by looking at them unblinkingly when you are making a powerful point or asking them to do something for you, just make sure it's not a confrontational look but a friendly one. This is achieved by simply smiling as you look. Below we will talk about some techniques.

Increase Your Status And Make People Feel As Though You Are Really Hearing Them

Focus on the eyes with a friendly smile so as not to seem threatening in a conversation, and you can focus on the eyes and then the points directly around the eyes, such as the eyebrow, the bone below the eye and to the sides of the eye. When most people are in a conversation, their eyes are going everywhere as they look around and think etc. By controlling your eyes, this will increase your status and make you seem more in control, it also gives the impression you are listening deeper which makes people like you, but it also causes the person to see you in a higher status and causes them to submit to you easier. Just make sure you are not staring in the eyes too long, make it natural, look at the eyes, then around the eyes and every so often look away. if you just focus on the persons eyes it will cause an uncomfortable feeling and will work against you.

Increase The Strength Of Your Request And Make Them Harder To Refuse

When you make a powerful point in your conversation or request something, you want to make direct eye contact, but again friendly. This makes your request much harder to say no to.

To Implant Your Thoughts Into Their Mind

During a conversation you can also look at the person's third eye and imagine the thoughts you want them to have, or the ideas you want them to agree with. This takes practice. Often when you're just starting out, it's a good idea to try to think of a subject and see if the person begins to talk about it, as an indication that your thoughts are being received. Also be aware that thoughts are transferable and anyone can do it, and the states of fascination and mesmerism make a person much more susceptible to picking them up.

To Influence The Subconscious Mind While In Conversation And Create Emotional Triggers

With this technique you can accomplish two things. You can influence the subconscious mind while talking directly to someone without them realizing it. This is great for influence and a sales situation, the other thing you can do is create an emotional trigger. This is where we create an emotion and then trigger the mind to remember that emotion on a cue. This is again great, as people often do things when they feel great or are happy.

While speaking to the person, look at their right eye and when you wish to say something you want the subconscious mind to be influenced by, switch to looking at their left eye. Consciously they will not realize it's being done but their subconscious will. The trick is to continue the process through the conversation. This will train the subconscious mind and begin to influence them. For example you could say "So (by now) I think (its time) to go to lunch". when you say the words in the parenthesis you would look at the left eye so the subconscious mind hears "buy now… its time) but the conscious mind only hears "by now it's time to go to lunch". This is a very subtle way of influencing and can be very powerful if done correctly.

You can also create emotional triggers, which allows us to subtly change the emotional state of a person with, in this case, just a look. As an example you can talk about regular things looking in the right eye and then when you say something funny or empowering, you look in the left eye. To set an emotional trigger It must be the same emotion each time. Eventually simply by looking in the left eye the person will feel the emotion automatically and will feel happy or ready to laugh, or empowered, which changes their mood and state.

To Seduce

While talking, you look slowly from the right eye to the left eye to the lips and back to the right eye. initially you do this for only about a second, slowing down your speech, but continuing to talk about the same non sexual subject you were, a moment ago and slowly making this triangle with your eyes. Then go right back to talking at the normal speed, and looking in their eyes as you would normally. After a few minutes you do this again, only taking about a second more, continue to do this slowly for longer and longer until you are doing it for about 5 seconds at a time. This will affect the other person as well, watch how they react. If they grow silent and lean in slightly or even look receptive, then when the time is right, you can make your move.

Different Types Of Gazes for Fascination

There are several types of gazes in fascination. Each has its advantages and techniques, which we will go over here.

1). The Basic Third Eye Gaze

This is the basic gaze and the one you will start out with. It will serve for most purposes. To do the gaze you look at the person's third eye, this is the space between their 2 eyes. Keep your eyes open wide as if in surprise, as you gaze unblinkingly. I personally find that if I can look at the person with the look and feeling of lust it helps, as it is a sexual energy, and at least for me it amplifies my fascination.

2). Right Eye Then Left Eye

This type of gaze can be used on someone to make them more submissive. The right eye is dominant and the left eye submissive. By focusing your gaze upon the right eye first and then the left eye it forces the brain to be more receptive and allows you to fascinate a difficult subject easier. This can also be used in conversations.

3). Rapid Eye Gaze

This is where your eyes dart quickly between the left and right eye and back. This confuses the mind and causes it to retreat within itself which is what we want.

4). Looking Through The Person

This gaze is when you look into their eyes and through them as if you are actually viewing something a foot or 2 behind their head. This causes your eyes to change focus and causes them to retreat into their mind putting them into fascination as well.

5). Distant Gaze

This is an old gypsy method. First you need to work on the right side of the person by either touching their right shoulder or shaking their right hand. This affects the brain. as the right side is controlled by the left side of the brain. You want to look at them as if you are looking far in the distance. Many times this technique will bring the person into trance with automatic movements.

1). Take the person's right hand as you look into their right eye, tell them to "imagine what you desire", or ask them "what is it you desire?"

2). Move your right hand and also your left one as this creates synchronicity.

3). Tell them to "look into my eyes and your desires will become true" then change your focus as if you are looking far off.

This will entrance the person at this moment.

6). Distant Gaze With Subtle Handshake

1). Shake the right hand and at the same time move your left hand, you can move it or place it on the person's arm you are shaking with the right hand.

2). Focus your eyes in the distance behind the person creating stupefied expression.

3). The subject will continue to move his hands in trance.

4). From here you can take the person to the floor, this works very quickly and subtly, but requires some practice to get it right.

It works because we are taking a normal everyday action and doing something unexpected with it, which throws the brain into confusion and then with the gaze the person succumbs to fascination quickly.

7). Using Eye Movement To Create Brain Hemisphere Dissociation

If we start concentrating on a person's eyes and alternate our gaze, starting from the right eye, and looking from one eye to the other we can cause hemispheric dissociation and help these techniques.

8). Distant Gaze With Suddenly Going Near The Persons Face

You use a distant gaze where you are focusing behind the person and move your head and eyes very close to the person suddenly, this can be very powerful and very good for healing.

9). *Effort And Vision*

1). Ask the person to place their palms on top of yours and push down with all their strength.

2). While the person does this there focus is absorbed.

3). Look quickly at the persons eyes, move your face and eyes very near them and begin to turn them around as you continue to fix your eyes on them.

4). The person will begin to follow you around with wide eyes as though attracted and fascinated and they will be unable to remove their eyes from you.

To Do Basic Fascination:

First if either you or the other person wears glasses make sure to take them off as the glasses distort the eye and will make the gaze more difficult. It does not matter if the person or you can not see well, remember this is about energy and they will feel the gaze regardless, even if their eyes are closed, but their eyes must not be distorted by glasses. You also want to open your eyes wider than normal, like a surprised look. As I mentioned earlier, I personally find that the feeling of lust gives more strength to the eyes, in addition you can imagine yourself making an EEEE sound this will cause your eyes to open wider and your face to adjust the way it should and it will also keep you in a more present state, because as you imagine this sound your mind will have more trouble wandering onto other subjects.

1). Put your left hand on their right shoulder this affects the left hemisphere of the brain and will help with fascination.

2). Look at the point between their eyes, at the third eye and take your fingers in the shape of a v and point at their eyes and bring them to your eyes, like a reverse Im watching you sign. This gives them a non verbal command to look into your eyes. It is important that you don't use words as words keep the conscious mind semi-active in order to be able to understand what you are saying. We want to shut the conscious mind down completely. By not using words you will find your trances are deeper and faster than regular hypnosis and have a higher success rate. You will be able to entrance about 95% of people with this technique compared to traditional hypnosis.

3). Begin to lightly sway with them just gently barely noticeable pushing and pulling them forward and back at the shoulder as you begin to use your right hand on the side of their face and move it in circular motion as you begin to draw them towards you with it, without touching their face.

4). Lift your left hand just barely off of them and see if they continue to sway as you sway with them mirroring them, as you watch them sway you can finally remove the left hand and just use your right hand.

5). Once they are in a state of fascination you can choose to keep their eyes open or close them depending on your needs. To close their eyes simply take your index and thumb and lightly touch their eyelids and draw them down. This light action helps bring them deeper. A fun way to do it is to also simply draw your hand down their face and watch their eyes close automatically. Once their eyes are closed, continue gazing at them for a moment or 2 longer. Do Not immediately change positions. It is interesting because even though they can't see you, they still feel your eyes gazing at them and it has an added effect.

6). Now you can mentally or verbally command them, or begin to do magnetism whichever you need.

You will know when they are in fascination by the look of their face. Their eyes will be wide open and unblinking. As you gaze at them, some people's blinking begins to slow, others will begin to speed up. On the people who's blinking begins to speed up, do not worry about it. This just means they are being affected differently, continue to gaze and you will see that promptly their blinking stops and their eyes stay open. You will also notice their face becomes expressionless. This happens because the muscles in the face relax. They will also continue to sway inexplicably or stay straight like statues a catatonic state.

In either state you can actually position their arms and hands in any position you want and they will keep them there. This is called catalepsy. In regular hypnosis this is a deep state and one that must be worked into, but in fascination and mesmerism because the techniques are non-verbal and energetic they are far more powerful and catalepsy it's actually the first state we will get, and it's very easy to get someone into. Incidentally in this state they can also not feel pain. We will talk more about this later when we talk about analgesia. It is possible to use these techniques as well to cause catalepsy and analgesia in the vocal cords so a person can not talk.

To Wake Them Up

There are several ways to wake someone up from fascination.

1). You can wave your hand in front of them as if you are fanning them as if they have fainted and this will wake them up, this is the classic way.

2). You can also give a short sharp blow of air with your mouth onto their face between the eyes. This is a very powerful way to wake a person.

3). You can take your index and thumb and massage the eyebrows starting at the bridge of the nose and going outward towards the outer edges of the eyebrows.

4). You can simply tap the side of the face gently and this will usually wake them if nothing else will.

A Note On Waking Up:

What I am about to say here is such a rarity that for most who read this book it will never happen in their entire lives. I only say it in the case that one day it may happen to one person somewhere, so that they are prepared and will not worry. This note applies more to Mesmerism, than fascination, but I have added it here on the off chance it may happen to you under fascination, that you will know what to do. Regardless of whether it happens in mesmerism or fascination the way to handle it is exactly the same.

It is very rare but there have been times where a person has not woken up with any technique. And while this is rare, if it should ever happen, simply stay calm, The subject will ALWAYS always wake. When this does happen most beginning Mesmerists are afraid that the person will stay in what's called the mesmeric sleep and not be able to wake, and will eventually die. You do not need to worry about this. The subconscious is always in control and will not allow them to stay in that state forever, or even to the point where their life will be in danger. What this generally means , on the rare occasions that a person does stay in the mesmeric sleep, is that the subconscious mind realizes it needs this state and sleep to heal more effectively, and so it stays in that state.

There was once a case of a person staying in the mesmeric sleep for 3 days, and even he woke up, and as the story goes, rather refreshed. If it does happen and a person refuses to wake, you have one more trick, you can speak to them and tell them that if they do not wake up, they may not (insert something very important to the person, or it could even be that you will not put them in this state again. etc.) If this does not work, simply move them to a comfortable place and let them stay, until they wake up on their own. Do not ever allow another person to try to wake them, unless they are a more skilled mesmer than you, as it can mix the energies and cause them to go deeper.

After you have mastered the basic fascination techniques you may begin to practice the more advanced ones below these are to be added to the basic technique to increase the power of your fascination.

ADVANCED TECHNIQUES TO IMPROVE AND DEEPEN FASCINATION

Faria Points

By first fascinating a person and then touching Faria points randomly and lightly you can re-equilibrate the body.

Faria was a Portuguese monk who originally discovered these energy points in the body. There are 2 ways to activate them. One is by direct touch and this is the strongest, but you can also almost touch them. By having the intention to touch and moving your hand close to the point but not touching it will still energetically activate the point. So if for some reason you can't touch the person this will be a good alternative option.

There are 2 reasons we use these points:

The First is for putting into trance. If you randomly touch these points after we get the person into fascination, you can cause the person to go deeper into trance faster. To use them for this, you only need to use the points above the waist. Touching them or almost touching them In a random order. The touches in this case are very short only for a second or so.

The second way they can be used is to help bring out the bad emotion or trauma for mesmeric crises therapy. Which we will talk more about later when we get into mesmerism.

The Faria Or Hypnogenic Points Are:

1). The Ankles

2). The Knees

3). The Thighs Above The Knees

4). The Belly

5). The Solar Plexus - one of the most important points

6). The Center Or The Chest

7). The Shoulders Between The Collar Bone

8). The Temple

9). The Third Eye

10). The Top Of The Head

11). The Back Of The Neck

Again to use them to increase trance we are going to randomly touch the belly, solar plexus, center of the chest, both the shoulders in the hollow hole felt just behind the collar bone, both the temples and the third eye.

A simple technique to eliminate general anxieties and fears is to ask the client where they feel an emotion, touch the different points, while gazing into their eyes and audible inhaling and exhaling.

Audible Breathing And Increasing And Decreasing Distance Suddenly

The last technique we will add is audible breathing. You want to have a loose expressionless face, this mimics what we want them to have, and as you do this open your mouth slightly and breathe in and out audibly, so they can hear you, this will increase the effects of the gaze and help them go into trance faster. In addition you can, while gazing, and breathing, quickly zoom in and away from their face with yours, this causes them to retreat into their mind. These last few techniques added to the ones above will make your fascination very strong.

Adding Passes

You can also use fascination and add in passes going down the persons arms as you gaze into them and this will also increase your fascination. You can learn the techniques for passes in the next section. When you notice the person is in fascination you can actually simply touch the third eye and slightly push and you will watch the person go backwards, make sure someone is behind them to catch them and take them to the ground and then from there you can do other things to heal them which we can discuss in the next chapter.

Fractionation

Fractionation is another technique that they use in traditional hypnotism. It was discovered that if you put someone into a trance that the next time you put them in, they go deeper, eventually it was discovered that you can put someone into a trance, bring them out and immediately put them in again and each time they will go deeper faster. We can use the very same technique with fascination and mesmerism as well. You simply gaze into their eyes and the minute they start to go into fascination, wake them, and then before they have fully come to, immediately begin to gaze and put them under again. Each time they will go deeper into the state. This can be useful for people that are resistant or difficult, or just for people that are not going deep enough.

Anesthesia With Fascination

By fascinating a person they will not feel pain, and so you can use this technique when someone is in pain, but also before a surgery or a dental procedure, or even labor. Before a procedure you must work with the person a few times and fascinate them so that they go deeper and get used to it. Simply fascinate them to the point of catalepsy, and then test by giving their arm a pinch etc and see if they respond. If they do you must continue to deepen the trance, if they don't, you have Anesthesia. Bear in mind that although a person can not feel, their body can still be damaged. I once saw a mesmerist use an open flame on a subject's foot, and while the subject felt nothing in trance his foot was still badly burned. So use tests that will not damage the client and with their permission, such as pinches, candle wax, etc.

Regression With Fascination

Fascination can be great for regressions. Regressions allow us to bring people back into the past, and will be discussed in more detail in a later chapter on Regressions.

1). Fascinate the person and with their eyes open.

2). You can use your arm to do a counterclockwise circle in front of the person then say when you drop your arm they will be at a point in time that was the first time they experienced x.

3). Then you begin to talk to them, and ask them if it is day or night, where they are, when they are, are they alone, or with someone etc. The process is fairly quick and can be interesting.

One more tip: As mentioned above, once in a fascinated state you can also give verbal commands such as to forget your name, 1+2=4 etc. like traditional hypnosis. While it is far better to use non verbal commands, this is something you can experiment with for fun should you want to.

Fascination Techniques To Use To Help Heal Yourself

Self Fascination Mirror Training

1). Go to the mirror, look at your left eye. Inhale and tense, exhale and relax.

2). Continue this, while always gazing into your left eye until you notice that your eye stays open without needing to blink very easily.

3). At this point stop, and turn around.

To Do Self Fascination and Self Hypnosis (Caduceus Exercise):

This is a very powerful technique to do self hypnosis and fascination and can be used to program yourself for whatever success you want.

Stand in front of a mirror, preferably a large mirror, if possible.

1). Stand Looking at yourself in the mirror between your eyebrows at your third eye. Try not to blink. Leave your arms at your sides, keep staring at your third eye, do this for about 30 seconds to 1 minute as you start to go into trance. You can make an EEE sound in your mind which will cause you to open your eyes wider the way they should be for fascination. While it is not necessary, it will help if you get the gaze correct.

2). Imagine your reflection as another person. Tell the other person in your mind to go backward, go backward, Stop, then go forward, go forward. Want the person to move in those directions and you will notice you move automatically in these directions. (this is very important as it's the basics once you can move back and forward you will be able to do everything else easier).

3). Then while looking at yourself in the mirror, tell the person in the mirror, your reflection, that your arms are light, and rising, rising (you will notice they begin to rise, it is not important how high they rise, only that they rise automatically).

4). Tell yourself you are nailed to the floor, nailed to the floor.

5). Feel a warmth in the solar plexus, as you do this.

6). Tell yourself in the mirror your gaze is very strong, or some positive affirmation you want to give yourself.

7). Tell yourself to turn around, then turn around and sit down.

(Chapter 2) Basic Mesmerism

As we mentioned in the intro, Mesmerism puts people in a healing trance but it is completely non verbal, and unlike hypnosis it almost always works. Because it is non verbal it is far stronger than regular hypnosis and you are not limited by language so it does not matter if they speak your language or not. In fact you can even entrance and heal from great distances. There is a lot you can do with Mesmerism.

In this section we will get you ready to do the basic Mesmeric induction. Just by putting someone into a mesmeric trance it will automatically help them remove blockages, help them heal from disease, or improve some area of their life they want to improve. The reason is when you are in a mesmeric trance the energy knows what it needs to do and will often do it without you as the practitioner having to do anything more advanced than just the basic induction. Just by learning this chapter you will be amazed at the kinds of results you can get. From healing people from pain that has caused them so much discomfort for years, to healing them from colds or headaches to helping them self improve from different issues they have. We will start with the basic exercises you need to master to be able to use mesmerism at its highest potential. While you will be able to use mesmerism without first practicing these exercises, I urge you to practice them as they will make all the difference, as you get more advanced.

Basic Essential Exercises

These next few exercises are critical to getting you ready to do magnetism and mesmerism at its highest level.

1). Breathing Exercise

This will give you an inner strength making your voice stronger and giving you more energy. It also opens up your ribcage which will increase your vitality and magnetic ability. You can do this 1-3 times a day to increase your energy.

- Inhale and bring your arms all the way up, making strong fists, then holding your breath you will bend over continuing to hold your breath, and keeping your muscles and fists tight, you continue to bend over bringing your arms parallel with your legs. in this position until you feel a sensation then come back up bringing your arms back straight up and then slowly exhale releasing your fists and slowly bringing your arms down.

2). Thymus Exercise

The Thymus is located directly behind the sternum in the center of the chest. Touching it increases energy and it also increases immunity due to the thymus gland located behind there as well. This will increase your magnetic strength over time.

- Put your arms up bent at the elbows, inhale, and as you inhale you move your arms back pushing your chest out so you feel the pressure on your thymus, tap your thymus, and hold your breath until you feel a sensation then blowout with force in 2 or 3 breaths moving your arms in circular motion.

Feeling Energy And Magnetism Exercise

These exercises are critical to begin feeling the energy of the body and being able to direct it. As well as feeling the energy of the other person's body.

3). Energy Sensation Exercise

Point a finger of one of your hands and then point it at the palm of your other and see if you can feel the sensation. As you begin to feel it you can experiment with distances on how far you can feel it.

4). Energy Ball Exercise

Place both palms together as if you are holding and invisible ball and feel the resistance. In the beginning it may help to rub your hands together first then place your hands to feel the energy easier. As you bring your hands closer you should begin to feel a slight resistance as if the energy or magnetic poles are repelling each other. As you continue to practice you will be able to feel the energy at greater and greater distances.

Advanced Exercise Once You Are Able To Induce By Passes

This exercise will increase your energy sensitivity.

Bring the person into a mesmeric state and perform magnetic passes. Stay in front of him, gazing in his eyes, thinking of the order "Go backward" Once they begin to respond and go backward on your unspoken command you are able to increase the difficulty by giving mental commands pushing and pulling the subject mentally.

BASIC PASSES

Now that you have worked on the exercises to increase your magnetic ability it's time to learn the basics of using mesmerism and to do that we will start by talking about passes.

Passes are the way you use your hands along a person's body to guide the energy. They are what allow you to entrance, and heal others. They work on everyone. With mesmerism you do not need to say a word and you can create very strong inductions. With Mesmerism you must feel the person and if your instinct says to focus on a particular area, focus on it. Mesmerism works, as long as they actually want help, this is important. When you do passes, you normally want to do them slow.

Everyone has a different definition of what this energy is being emitted is, with the passes, and with mesmerism, some say it's a mesmeric fluid others say it's a type of electricity. I myself feel it is a mesmeric fluid, an ether that flows from us. However if you read the books of the past everyone has a different explanation and definition, and the truth is mankind as a general rule, always wants to define, because we don't like not knowing. But isn't this what Magick and the Divine are, are they not the secrets of nature. How can the finite ever truly comprehend the infinite. I tell my students don't get lost in the theories of the past. Visualize it how you want to because that is what will allow you to use it.

It helps to have a visualization, so I will tell you what we do seem to know and what everyone does agree on. We can look at this as an energy that flows from the palms of the hands and fingers, eyes, and even the mouth. It has similar properties to electricity, there is a positive and negative and often the energy must be grounded and balanced which we will talk about later. when we use our hands or even our eyes, or mouth, there is a mesmeric fluid that comes out from it. An energy that flows, and it has been said that some who are sensitive are even able to see this essence being emitted from the fingers and hands of the practitioner.

It is important to know that the energy comes from the part of the hand with the palms and not the back of the hand-. So when we do passes we go in the direction we want with our palms and fingers facing the person then turn the back of our hands towards the person before going back to the starting position. Because if we were to just go up and down with the palms facing the person, then on one stroke it would magnetize, and on the return stroke it would de-magnetize and so the person would never feel any effect.

Types Of Passes

There are many types of passes, each has its purpose which are discussed below, but don't get overwhelmed. The most basic ones are the longitudinal passes which you will use in the beginning the most.

Longitudinal-Passes - These are passes made in a longitudinal manner, i.e., lengthwise over the body; For example from the head to the solar plexus.

Transverse-Passes - These are passes made across the Subject's body, as from shoulder to shoulder.

Right Transverse passes - These are made from the Operator's right to left.

Left Transverse-passes - These are made from the Operators left to right.

Reverse-Passes or Demagnetizing-Passes - These are used to remove the effect of the last Magnetising-Passes, and are done in a quicker opposite direction. From bottom the body towards the top.

Local or Topical-Passes - These are made over any specific area, such as the persons Solar plexus, head, or hands.

Frictions or Stroking's - These are passes with contact, and are named after the passes, for example:

Longitudinal-frictions, or Transverse-frictions

These next 2 Passes are used a lot in Fascination:

Drawing-Passes - These are used for the purpose of attracting or drawing Subjects towards you.

Repelling-Passes - These are used to make Subjects move away from you and are done in the reverse way of the drawing passes.

Bridges - Bridges are not passes they are a way of balancing energy between two points, but are very important and this is the best place to mention them. When doing a bridge you will place one hand on one energy point in the body and the other on another point and this bridges the 2 points balancing the energy between them. This is useful for pain and energy balancing and we will mention when to use them in techniques below.

Pyramids - Pyramids are made by placing your hands so that both thumbs and both forefingers touch and the space between both hands creates a pyramid. Your palms ofcourse facing the person. Pyramids can be used to focus energy.

Inverse Pyramids - This is done in the same way as a regular pyramid, except you're making an upside down triangle.

Downward slow passes are used to relax and put a person into a trance, upward quick passes are used to bring energy back to the person and bring them out of trance, which is used to wake them up.

When you do passes, You must feel calm and look at the person as you do this. It is also important that you are using presence while you work with the subject, this keeps your mind from daydreaming and you will be in the here and now, and this is where you will have more ability and power with magnetism and mesmerism.

Important notes: The subject feels what you feel, in fact once in trance you can walk a few paces away, change your breathing rate and you will see the subject also changes theres to match yours. So keep these points in mind as work.

1). You must feel calm

2). Feel no pressure, just see what happens and watch as it does.

Basic Self Passes On Yourself

This technique will allow for self-hypnosis and self-healing.

1). Sit in a comfortable chair and take your right hand and do longitudinal passes over your left side stopping at your solar plexus. To do passes simply take your hand and slowly go down your body, not touching the body but close to it. So you can feel the energy. Then do the same thing with your left hand over the right side of the body. Continue to do this for 3 or 4 times and you will feel a sensation, make sure you are doing this balanced on both sides of the body.

You can also use the charges technique we talk about below, for yourself instead of using passes.

How To Work With People

There are 4 steps to hypnosis and mesmerism:

1). Never magnetize someone who is testing you or does not really want it. While the non-verbal techniques are much more powerful than regular hypnosis, why work with someone that isn't serious about being healed or is trying to show you up.

2). You must have the person concentrate in his mind what they want to achieve by the mesmeric process. This can be accomplished by first asking them what it is they would like to improve, this can be a physical pain, an illness, or some mental issue or even stress or self improvement they would like to accomplish.

3). Put them in a a mesmeric state with the passes.

4). Once they are in this state they will automatically change and improve whatever it was they wanted to work on, it will also just by being in a trance have a healing effect on their body whether their condition is caused by disease or pain.

INDUCTIONS

Now we are going to talk about how to use this information to induce people into trance, and this is where the fun, and healing begins. Interestingly enough as you begin to strengthen your abilities your energy will naturally strengthen and so by learning to heal others you will begin to find that you yourself are healed as well.

How To Do Mesmerize A Person Standing

When you do mesmerism with a person standing you will want them to go to the floor and they will go, but often you will need to tell them beforehand that when this happens that you will catch them. You can also have them fall backward into your arms like you would a trust exercise first, while they are still awake, and this will teach their subconscious that you will catch them. If you dont you can still do everything but in the beginning you will find the person's subconscious mind will not allow them to fall back. It wants them to be safe so you will see they start to fall back but then they will catch themselves, almost wake up, and right themselves, then go back into trance. And you want them to end up on the floor as this deepens the trance and aids in healing. So after you explain and do the trust exercise...

There are 2 ways to start.

The 1st is to use fascination on them first, and after they are in fascination, you can just close their eyes by using your index and thumb to draw their eyelids shut. This is the more powerful technique, and one of the quickest ways to get them into mesmerism.

The 2nd option is weaker and slower but will still work. WIth this option you simply just close the persons eyes using your thumb and finger and then begin using passes without doing fascination first.

I will always suggest you use fascination first, always. This is because not only does fascination greatly increase the speed at which you can get someone into trance but it also increases the depth of the trance and increases the persons ability to be healed in that session. So its a far stronger method and super easy, but regardless of which option you choose, the next steps are below.

1). In the beginning, when you first start out, you can start by rubbing your 2 hands together quickly so that you feel a vibration or ants between them. This allows you to feel the energy a little easier in the beginning when you are just starting. Later after you begin to develop your ability to feel energy you won't need to do this.

2). Stand to the side of the person and place your 2 hands one infront of the person's head at their forehead and the other behind their head at the base of the skull. Hold your hands close and relaxed but make sure your hands are not straight and flat but curved as if holding a ball and relaxed. This is important because if your hands are straight and tight this will close off the energy and it will not flow like it needs to from your hands. You want your hands close and almost touching them but still some space between your hands and their head.

3). You can Imagine an energy between your two hands, and visualize it going through the person. And very slowly bring your hands down the length of the person, the one in front staying in front and the one behind them staying behind them both moving down slowly together. As you notice the person start to sway or have some reaction, even a slight one, stop there at that point and wait for a moment, until the reaction stops then continue.

4). You will continue down and stop at the solar plexus area and hold your hands there for a moment, this will deepen the trance, and cause the person to go into somnambulism. While your hands are there and still facing the solar plexus area you can move both your hands about 30 cm away from the body and then bring them back to the original distance. This helps concentrate the energy at the solar plexus. This is considered 1 pass. You will want to make at least 3 or 4 passes to bring the person into trance.

5). Once you hold your hands over the solar plexus for a moment, you pull your hands away, and move them back to the starting position on the top of the person's head. Make sure that as you raise your hands back to the top of the head again, that as you move your hands back up, your palms are not facing the person. Because this will undo what you just did. When you move your hands back up to the top of the head you want to turn your hands out and away so the back of your hands are facing the person, or simply close your fingers into a very loose fist as you go up to the head. Then repeat the same process and this will deepen the trance.

6). As you continue you will notice the person is swaying more and more and will almost appear to be falling over. In most cases their subconscious will not allow them to fall but you should always be ready to catch them if they do. When they look as if they can barely stand, simply go behind them and a slight very gentle pull from behind on their forehead will be enough to topple them into your arms. It will be only a feather touch of pressure to cause them to fall back.

7). Once the person is flat on the floor, you do not need a pillow, a flat surface works best, you will put your thumb and middle finger of the same hand on each of their temples as you grasp and lightly move their head from side to side, this deepens the trance. You can then do some circular movements over the solar plexus and you can then use Farea points again if you wish. You will always after this use longitudinal passes down their entire body, 2 or 3 times this deepens. You can also take both your hands, one on each side of the person's head, over the temple area, and then move them in a circular movement a few times without touching the head. This is a very strong deepener as well. At this point you could do more advanced work, or give them verbal hypnotic commands, or in this case since we are just mastering the basic induction simply let them stay in this state for a bit to heal and when it comes time you can wake them up. They do not need to be in this state long, 10-15 minutes is usually enough to heal most minor things.

To Mesmerize Someone Sitting

1). Have both you and the subject sit on a chair facing each other. Place the person's knees between your knees. So your knees are touching theirs.

2). Have them make a thumbs up by closing their fists with the thumbs up bent at the arms.

3). Grab their hands and touch your thumbs to their thumbs and gaze into their eyes. hold their thumbs and then after a few minutes slowly pull your hands away and see if they keep their hands in place.

4). If they start to drop their hands keep holding them until when you slowly pull away their hands stay in the same location. until they stay held in the air without moving. This is called catalepsy.

5). Then you can close their eyes and continue to gaze into their eyes, and do downward passes down the front of their body and stop at the solar plexus.

Induction With Light

1). Have the person look at the light, and focus only on the light and nothing else you can also look at the light for a moment to help you get into the right state of mind.

2). Have them breath deeply, breath audible for them.

3). Do some passes over the solar plexus by keeping the hands over the solar plexus but pulling them farther away and bringing them closer to the solar plexus. you can also do light touching on the upper faria points this helps check for degrees of relaxation, and have the left hand pass slightly behind the base of the head. You will be able to verify that the subject is letting go.

4). At this point you can put the subject on the ground and close their eyes in the usual way.

5). You can also verbally tell them to relax and let go.

The ground will actually deepen the state and You can put an arm in catalepsy, to see how deep they are. Or, you can deepen and do a regression, which we will cover later.

Eliminating The Senses

This is with the idea of taking each sense and drawing it down to the solar plexus taking these senses away, and the movement is done fairly quickly. This is a quick way to put people back in trance after they have already been there. And this can be very useful if you want to work on yourself as well, as doing passes on yourself can be a little difficult. So it can be the equivalent of doing passes. To do this technique you will use both hands at the same time.

1). Take your 2 thumbs and put them on top of their head and pull down over their face towards the solar plexus like you are drawing their spirit there. Do this 3 times.

2). Take your 2 index fingers and place them at the eyes and draw them down over the face towards the solar plexus. Do this 3 times.

3). Take your 2 middle fingers and place them at the persons ears and draw them towards the front of the face and then down over their face and towards the solar plexus. Do this 3 times.

4). Take both your ring and pinky fingers and place them on each side of the face along the jaw as to be close to the nose and mouth and draw towards the front of the face and then down over the face and onto the solar plexus. Do this 3 times.

After you finish these movements you can then put the hand on the solar plexus to deepen the trance. You can further deepen by putting one hand on the solar plexus and the other on the occiput at the base of the head, and then afterwards bringing that hand down and placing it on the persons back right behind the solar plexus while the other hand stays in front of the solar plexus.

REMOTE INDUCTIONS

The Remote Induction

This induction is based on the principle of the difficulty that the subject has when he tries to follow the practitioners hand and pay attention to the practitioners eye at the same time.

This method works very well for zoom etc., but not so well in real life.

1). Hold your hand up, palm facing them.

2). Ask them to put their hand facing yours and follow the movement of your hand with theirs. Tell them to follow your hand with theirs as you move it randomly rocking back and forth toward the screen. Continue to tell them to follow your hand as you breath heavily, then say LOOK at me, (use the fascination gaze as you look at them, Looking at the camera son on their screen your eyes will be facing theirs) As you say to look at me, move your hand to the side so they have trouble looking at your hand and your eyes) Then continue again and say follow my hand, look at my eyes. Continue to do this over and over until they go into trance. You will notice they start to have trouble following your hand, it usually takes a few minutes to get them into trance.

The Hand Induction

This can be done remotely or in person. There are 4 main points to be aware of with this induction

1). You want to have the person concentrate on their stomach and the air filling it.

2). They have to have trust you as they do with all hypnosis.

3). Have them take deep breaths (show them how to breath like when a doctor is checking your chest you make those deep loud breaths this is the same here).

4). Let them know that when you tell them to move their head during the induction they will move their head from left to right (show them by you turning your head from left to right).

Have the person put their hand up as if they are making a promise, close their eyes and start to breathe as they breathe to, tell them to notice the air filling their stomach. Tell them you will count back from 10-1 and the dream will begin.

The hypnotist should take deep audible breaths as he counts this helps the subject go down. You can say similar things as are listed here as you count down. 10 the air filling your stomach, 9 breath, 8, 7 air entering, and going down, 6, 5 while you make breathing sounds, tell them to move their head left to right. 4, Tell them "if your hand wants to stay there it is okay if it wants to fall that is okay too." 3, 2 breathing, 1 and the dream can begin.

From here you can give them positive suggestions, suggest a regression, or make them hear or see things like in a dream.

A good sign to look for is if their hand stays up this is a sign of catalepsy which we will cover later but it indicates they are in a state, but if it doesn't stay up, that is okay too.

Charges

This is a way of using passes from a distance when you can't use them in person such as on zoom or the phone. This is also a great way of doing passes on yourself, as you will find it easier than doing physical passes. This is also good for insomnia, and to use for the practitioner to get used to being present and feeling their body. Oftentimes when a technique like the ball of light does not work well remotely you can then use charges and most of the time after it should be fine.

To Do The Technique:

1). Have the person close their eyes, and inhale, feel their feet then exhale.

2). Inhale, then feel their legs, exhale.

3). Inhale, feel their lower torso, exhale.

4). Inhale, feel their torso, exhale.

5). Inhale, feel their head and arms, exhale.

6). Repeat, the cycle 1 or 2 times.

7). Then count 123 and have them open their eyes.

Once you do a regular induction with fascination and passes, sometimes you can walk away a short distance and it will allow the person to have a type of reaction that may be different for each person so you will just have to observe and see what happens. An experiment you can do when you walk away, is to purposely change your breathing rate, and you will notice the subject should change theirs to match yours automatically, even if they can't see you. Sometimes if you stay with the person too much it can block them. If they have the reaction you can then go back and do more passes or continue to work on them, if they don't have a reaction after a short time you can still go back and continue.

NON VERBAL INDUCTION

To use this technique simply put the person in the center of the room. Close their eyes, and begin to walk around them in a circle, making noise with your feet. As you do so you can use the Faria points to touch or lightly randomly touch different parts of their upper body to induce the trance more. In addition you can talk to them in inaudible or unintelligible words. Words that have no meaning It is very useful to use the phrase dos, for example.

You can test them by seeing if there is catalepsy by placing their hand in a certain position and see if it stays there. You can also use HUH sounds like the goose sound, clicking sounds with your mouth. Once they are standing there in trance you can verbally command the person like regular hypnosis. Maybe you want them to go to the floor and have someone waiting to catch them. Then you can tell the unconscious, "unconscious, push him backward" etc.

Once you get them on the ground you will touch the solar plexus and do passes over the body, and then begin to work from there.

Energisation

This is a very easy and very powerful technique. It alone can be used to put a person in a magnetic state. And it's very subtle so you don't even need to mention magnetism. It also allows the person to be more reactive to the energy.

To Do Energisation

1). Put your hands on the person's ankles and hold them there.

2). Have the person's arms touching the sides of them with their eyes closed and ask them if they feel an energy going up for their legs. (this activates the parasympathetic nervous system when they feel the sensation within them.

3). When they say or nod yes, tell them to let the energy continue going up their leg through their body to their head. and once it gets to the top of their head, have them feel it traveling back down to their feet.

After a moment or so you will notice they begin to go into a state of magnetism.

SUBTLE INDUCTION

This is a slightly more advanced technique but still very easy. It allows you to induce a person without even mentioning magnetism.

First you must do energisation.

Once you have done the energisation you then feel the left palm and feel the heat, then do the same with the right palm, if you feel one is colder than the other send energy into it, without touching it.

Then go to the person's head put one hand in the front of the forehead and one in the back at the occiput to begin the trance state

Once you have held your hands here for a few moments you then go behind the person and put your hands over the top of their head. One hand over the right side of the brain, the other over the left side of the brain. As you do this the person will slip into a magnetic trance deeper and deeper

Energy Chi Ball

You can do magnetism with yourself by using the energy chi ball in front of the chakra you want to work on and activate. This is done by holding an imaginary energy ball and manipulating it as if rolling a volleyball in front of the energy center you wish to work on. Imagine your energy mixing with the energy ball and being completely renewed and changed.

To Wake Them Up

You have several options:

1). Quick upward passes as if fanning them.

2). You can take your fingers and rub the eyebrows.

3). You can blow on the face.

4). You can tap them on the side of the face

5). But you can also do something pretty cool and speak to the subconscious mind. You can give them all kinds of commands like in normal hypnotism. One of the more fun ways to wake a person is to call the person by their name. Tell them that they may remain in this sleep until they are done, but they must wake by a certain time, within 30 minutes or at a specific time as an example, say 2pm. If they do not answer, you may ask them, do you understand, and get confirmation. What's really interesting is even though their eyes are closed and they can not see a clock, you will find they wake within a minute or 2 of the time you mentioned.

Once they wake up, you can close the session, or you can also do an immediate induction again, and get them to go even deeper into trance the next time. This is the same as fractionation with verbal hypnosis, which we will discuss a little later.

MAGNETIC ATTRACTION

This is an incredibly fun way of getting people to fall back or forward. You can have a person follow your hands once they are in trance as if you are pulling them by an invisible connection. This is for more advanced things such as clairvoyance, or telepathy and not so much for healing or therapy. But you can use the forward pull we will talk about for therapy.

In either case you can do these magnetic pulls by simply putting your hands in front of them about chest level and pulling your hand back imagining them being pulled by your hand and you will see them follow as if an invisible string is pulling them. You can do the same thing from behind and pull them backward as well. The best place to do these backward pulls from behind is on a person's back right between the shoulder blades or at the base of the skull. The forward pulls you can do from the center of the person's chest. You can, also with practice, do forward pushes in this way.

As you get stronger and stronger with this technique you can begin to attract other parts of their body and even make them follow you, walking towards you with almost superhuman strength. Just by bringing your hand near the arm of the magnetized subject you will watch his arm go out to you and follow all your hands movements. People that go into somnambulism easily are called somnambules and this ability of magnetic attraction is possessed by many somnambules, and it can be grown and improved. Little by little the magnetized person becomes more sensitive to various movements and attractions, and if you add a quick understanding of gestures to this then the magnetized subject appears to be being controlled by your mind. In reality it eventually becomes unconscious communication between the magnetized and the mesmer. In the beginning a person can only understand simple movements at close distances, but in time he understands the magnetizer and his gestures and he will follow almost unnoticeable directions from the mesmer.

Also the phenomenon of bodily attraction can be produced by merely the presence of the magnetizer and can be improved by the mesmer's mental thoughts or even just created by it. Magnetic attraction and magnetic rapport can be done at greater distances once you are able to do it at close distance.

Ways To Do Magnetic Attraction With Palms Of Your Hands

Attraction With The Gaze

Look into the person's left eyes, fascinating them and then use your hands on both sides of their head and do a drawing forward motion as you mentally command them to come forward. You will shortly watch them sway forward towards you.

The Energetic Pull

After you do passes and put the person into a state,

1). Put your 2 open hands on the shoulders of a person's back. You can begin by touching the person's back right at the shoulder blades.

2), Then pull your hands away and keep them about 50mm and stay like this.

3). Imagine your warmth and energy mixing with their warmth and energy.

4). Slowly pull your hands back as if you are pulling them, and you will see they go back with you. If in the beginning they do not go back immediately but sway back and stop, it is okay, simply move your hands into position again about 50mm and pull back again, until they fall backward into your arms.

The Invisible Cord Technique

Once they are in a state,

1). Make the person close their eyes, touch their eyelids as you close them.

2). Go behind the person, imagine grabbing a cord right in the middle of their shoulder blades. You can use both hands and just pull back. And intend that they fall back. You may have to pull the cord and then go back to the starting position and pull them again to get them to fall back. Once you get used to it you can do it from a distance as well. The amazing thing is that it doesn't matter if the person sees you or not, they respond to your energy and intention. If you want to pull them forward just pull the invisible string from the front sternum area.

(Chapter 3) Helping The Physical Healing Of Pain And Disease

The techniques below are more specific than just the general mesmeric trance we have talked about up to this point. These techniques will allow you to help a person heal from sickness, disease, pains, and physical damage to the body. Understand that, as we have previously mentioned, just by putting someone into a mesmeric trance they will begin the healing process, but the steps below will take your healing to the next level. Depending on the severity of the issue it may take one session or multiple. The one rule with mesmerism is to always make sure that if you decide to help someone heal, and if they have a severe disease, you are willing to see it through until the end, even if that may take months or longer. If you are not willing to do this or can not, then do not help them.

How To Conduct A Healing Session

First speak to the person and ask them if they really want help. If someone doesn't really want help then don't treat them. Sometimes people will say they want help or their friends or relatives will, and you will see that the person is fighting and resisting going into trance. At this point I would just stop and ask them if this is something they really want and speak to them a little, if it is and they are just nervous that is one thing, but again if they are not really wanting help. It's not worth your time, because you can not do anything if their body does not want to be helped, remember it is them that is healing themselves you are just facilitating, and if they don't want to heal you can be the best mesmer in the world and it won't matter. There are 4 general steps depending which technique below you prefer.

1). Talk to the person, find out what is wrong, find out if they want to heal, and make them feel at ease and comfortable. In this step you will explain what you are going to be doing and make sure they feel good, a joke here helps.

2). A magnetic diagnostic.

3). Induction.

4). The end steps to wake and give them magnetic water.

To Do A Diagnostic:

This will allow you to feel where there is an energy blockage. So that you can begin working on this area. Move the hand down the back without touching along the spine: the client will move where the hand passes at the location where the pain or trouble is. To treat this area you can put your hands in a triangle position with fingers pointing to the painful zone.

Treatment Time Breakdown

When you do a treatment the general time should be about 18-20 minutes, normally about 2 minutes for rapport and induction, 15 minutes for treatment, and 3 minutes to let them rest and come back.

To do a treatment there are several techniques available but these 2 below are fairly easy and very effective.

Method 1: The Original Mesmer Method

1). Have the client speak about the problem.

2). Look into their eyes and fascinate them while you do stroking passes down their arms.

3). Touch the solar plexus.

4). Touch or concentrate over the point of pain.

Method 2: The Puysegur Method

This was the method that the Marquis de Puysegur, a follower of Mesmer used.

1). Talk to the client about the problem.

2). Do a Magnetic Diagnosis.

3). Do a Magnetic Induction.

4). Focus energy on the solar plexus and use Faria points. The solar plexus is a very strong point, by focusing the energy on this area you are working on the enteric nervous system. and bringing them into somnambulism.

5). Once the person is in a somnambulistic state, work on the part that is causing the sickness or pain.

6). At the end you can use magnetic water to finish the procedure which helps and you can show them how to do it for themselves as well. We will cover this a little later.

A Word On Somnambulism

Somnambulism is a dream type state that can allow people to talk and react but still be in trance. This is the 3rd stage a person goes into in Mesmerism. The 1st we have already talked about being Fascination. The 2nd being Catalepsy which we will talk about in a moment, the 3rd somnambulism, and the 4th is lethargy which is a state where the person's body is completely limp and unresponsive, we won't go too much into this last stage except to explain it so you may know what stage a person is in when you see this.

Going back to somnambulism,It's an interesting state because in somnambulism a person seems to have access to unconscious knowledge. In the past, a mesmer might bring someone into a somnambulistic state and then ask them questions about their disease or issues, and the person having access to the subconscious mind would be able to say what they had, whether the mesmer would be able to help them or not, and exactly what they would need to heal. Often having no memory of the conversation afterwards when they were awakened.

However please note that we should not be doing this as its diagnosing and only a doctor can truly do this. In addition if it does happen accidentally while a person is in a trance and they begin to tell you things, you should never just take a somnambulist's word on a healing procedure, but must ALWAYS verify with their doctor if it could really help them or not. In such cases you may write down the suggestion the somnambulist gives and then give it to them when they awaken and have them check with their doctor. To see if it is something that could help.

In addition, in the somnambulistic state people seem to be able to have esp and psychic abilities, often knowing what objects are hidden under clothes or where in a room they were hidden, and seem to have heightened senses and are able to hear and smell things that could not possibly be heard or smelt by a normal person in a normal state. There are many very interesting experiments done with somnambulists that I would recommend looking further into, reading up on, and trying. It is interesting to note that not all people are somnambulistic and some will bypass this stage.

Also please know that you do not need to use these kinds of tricks when using the Puysegur method, though they can be fun for experimenting, simply putting them in a somnambulistic state and working on them is enough.

USING MESMERISM FOR ANESTHESIA AND PAIN RELIEF

Catalepsy And Anesthesia

This is the 1st state you can achieve in Mesmerism and it is very easy. When you fascinate a person or mesmerize them you will notice there comes a point where their arms are just staying in the air. There are 2 kinds of catalepsy, the 1st is a freezing of the body and immobility, such as when you hear a strange sound and freeze to figure it out. This is a milder state. The 2nd state is immobility, and completely being frozen with fear, though it is not just fear it is when the deeper mind takes over eliminating the conscious mind. This can happen naturally with traumatic events.

When we get a person into catalepsy with trance you will find the state builds upon itself. You can take a person's arm and straighten it out and they will hold it in position, once you get one arm in position, you can then put the other in position, and then a leg, then the other leg, and eventually the whole body can be positioned in different positions and the person will keep it there often with great strength as if the limb has been locked into place. There are many demonstrations of placing a person's feet on one chair and their head on another and nothing beneath the rest of the body. The catalepsy is so strong that their body stays perfectly rigid and people can even sit on their body and it will not bend. Though I don't recommend doing this. while they will not bend we don't want to cause damage to their body or injure them. Remember we are healing. I only mention it here to show how strong the catalepsy is and how interesting the phenomenon is. When you wish to unlock the limbs you will find it's very easy. Just grab the limb and shake it slightly side to side and this will unlock it and the person will allow you to bring it back down.

This is an interesting experiment but what is even more interesting is the fact that when a person is in catalepsy they also do not feel pain in the region. It creates anesthesia, to such a degree that whole medical surgeries have been performed on a person where they felt nothing. It is important to note that you do not need to have the limb cataleptic to have anesthesia but often they go hand in hand. You can test this by putting a person into catalepsy and pinching their arm or even pouring hot candle wax on their hand and you will notice they do not feel it. You must be careful though because even though they do not feel it they can still be damaged so don't put a flame directly to their skin while they may not feel it it will still burn the tissue.

In fact there was a Dr Esdaile who worked in India and was famous for using mesmerism to cause anesthesia, not only would he perform major surgeries without the people feeling it, but they bled less and recovered quicker with less infection. He would also raise one arm up and know that if it lowered the person was coming out of trance so he could use this as a way of monitoring their state. He wrote a very interesting book on it called "Mesmerism in India and its Practical Application in Surgery and Medicine by James D Esdaile. M.D." and I would recommend anyone to look it up and read it if they get a chance.

Analgesia

These techniques have been used to prevent pain like before a surgery, and also to remove pain that is already there. When you have muscular tensions, and skeletal pain, it is good to use analgesia to remove the pain, but you also want to solve the cause of the pain as well. Also by learning to create analgesia it can be a turning point in mesmerism, and fascination, because once you get them in analgesia it causes the people to respond better to all other techniques, such as telepathic techniques, and hypno-mentalism.

Local Analgesia

So now you know how you can create whole body anesthesia, as it happens almost automatically with a mesmeric trance and catalepsy, but what if you only need to heal pain in certain areas without putting people in a cataleptic state. The next few techniques will teach you how to do that.

To create local Anesthesia there are several techniques:

Using Passes On Yourself Or Another

1). Do passes, away from the body towards the ends of the extremity on the part that needs the anesthesia.

2). Go slowly and the area will begin to feel a tingling and a loss of feeling.

3). To test this you can try to pinch the area where you have the tingling sensation and should notice a reduction in feeling. Or if you are working on another person, they should feel a reduction in pain.

Counter Clockwise Circles

With general pain you can decrease it by doing counterclockwise circles over the area affected. Just hold your hand slightly above the area and do a counterclockwise circle making sure to stay present. This is very effective and works very quickly. It can be done on someone else or even yourself if you have pain.

Bridges

Bridges are very useful in mesmerism and allow you to connect 2 energy points at the same time, This balances the energy and regulates them. Allowing you to remove pain and help heal the body.

To do a bridge place one hand over one energy point like the third eye and the other hand on another energy point like the solar plexus and so you are bridging these two points and this will regulate the energy between them, when you make a bridge you just touch and hold it for about 30 seconds or until you feel the points are balanced before moving on. You can systematically bridge each point in the body and this will be great for overall energy balancing.

To Make A Bridge For Pain

As an example, if a person has a pain on the left side:

1). Put them in a magnetic trance.

2). Put your hand on the side without the pain first.

3). Put your other hand on the other side with pain.

4). This will bridge the 2 parts and balance the energy; this will remove the pain.

Erminio Di Pisa's Technique

This is an incredibly fast and effective way of eliminating pain in seconds. It was used by a famous healer named DI Pisa who was famous in Italy for rapid pain relief. This can be used for pretty much any pain relief, and for difficulties moving as well.

1). You as the practitioner must believe you can do this.

2). Ask the person where the pain is, and on a scale of 1-10, how strong is the pain.

3). Next you touch or have the person touch where the pain is.

4). Make sure the person is open, you can tell a joke, or just make sure they are comfortable

5). Tell them to look right at your third eye, and Begin to use fascination on them.

6). Once they begin to go into fascination, blow at the point between their eyes suddenly, and quickly move your hand or have them move theirs from the injured area as if you are sweeping the pain away.

7). Take both hands and grab the sides of their head placing your thumbs gently but firmly over their closed eyes and rotate the head in a circular motion 3 times.

This should eliminate the pain but if not you can always do a second round.

Earaches

To work with an earache it's important to know that the mesmeric fluid flows from not only our fingers and eyes, but also our breath. So you can take a linen cloth and place it on the affected ear, open your mouth and breathe out slowly onto the ear so that your hot breath penetrates through the cloth into the ear. This usually begins to work very quickly.

Headaches

Technique 1

To help with headaches simply put one hand on the occiput or base of the skull and the other on the forehead. You can either place your hands right on the areas or hold them a few inches away. And simply hold your hands in this position for about 20 seconds as you visualize yourself being grounded and the energy flowing from your hands and their head down to the ground.

Technique 2

Make a bridge from the forehead to the thymus and hold it there for about 20 seconds.

How To Eliminate Personal Pain

Mirror Technique

1). Look at yourself in the mirror between the eyes. Don't blink.

2). Tell yourself go backward come forward go backward come forward.

3). Tell yourself your arms are light and they are rising. continue as you watch your arms begin to rise.

4). Bring your hands down, Look at yourself in the right eye, inhale, hold your breath and tighten all of your muscles, then exhale and relax. Do this several times.

5). Then Look at your left eye, inhale, hold your breath and tighten all of your muscles,then exhale and relax. Do this several times.

6). Now look at your right eye and pay attention to your body, to your heart, and feel yourself in your body.

7). Begin to inhale, pay attention to your heart and feeling it more and more, and at the same time open your arms like chicken wings, inhale and inhale filling your lungs completely, then breath out, and begin to move your arms and hands in a circular forward motion in a similar way as telling someone to come on, or hurry up, as you completely empty your lungs.

8). Touch your solar plexus, and begin to do it all over again. Do this several times.

9). On the final exhale, when you touch your solar plexus you should feel less or no pain.

(By emptying your lungs in the manner above as well as touching your solar plexus it stimulates the parasympathetic system, and can allow you to eliminate pain from yourself.)

Remote Techniques

The Ball Of Light

This technique is good for Zoom and Skype, or can be used on the phone as well

1). Have the person look at you or listen to you and put one hand on the place where the pain is.

2). Tell them to breathe, open your mouth slightly and use fascination, or another induction as you begin to breathe out loud.

3). Tell them to continue looking at you or listening to you.

4). Tell them now, to imagine a ball of light coming from above the body and it is now entering their body. This light is warm and light, interrupt this by telling them to look into your eyes, or listen to you etc. Then again, tell them this light is warm and light, and the warmth goes where it is needed. or a version similar.

5). Have them quickly move their hand.

6). Count 123 and have them close their eyes... then after 1 or 2 seconds have them open their eyes. Tell them to turn their head, (show them to turn their head left and right in both directions. Then ask them, how do they feel now?

GENERAL THERAPIES

These general therapies are very good for regulating the body over all, they can be done by themselves or for a more powerful healing effect, they can be done all together depending on what is wrong with the person. The steps below are after you have put the person into a magnetic state.

Remember that below you will see a lot of bridging. To do the bridge connect the two energy points like mentioned, and then wait about 30 seconds or until you feel those two points are balanced, before moving on to the next bridge in the series for that treatment. Do not immediately move from point to point like the techniques have been written. The techniques below can be used for another person or can be used on yourself, for self healing.

For self fascination you will need to use the mirror and when it mentions passes you may do the self passes discussed above, or if it requires long passes down the body, you may use the charges in their place, as this is great to move the energy just like passes but easier when working on ourselves.

1. For General Pains

1). Bridge the front part of the head with the thymus.Do this until you feel it's time to move on.

2). Bridge the thymus with the solarplexus.

3). Bridge the liver with the spleen.

2. For Immunitary And To Increase Energy

1). Bridge the Thymus and the Spleen and liver area.

2). Bridge the occiput with the tailbone.

3). Bridge the occiput and push energy into the left and right armpit one at a time. (You can do this by taking your free hand and fanning or pushing energy towards the left armpit area several times before moving to the left armpit area) Next continue to bridge the occiput but put energy into the outer left and right sides of the groin one at a time, in the same manner as above.

3). To Revitalize

1). Bridge the head and thymus.

2). Bridge the thymus and solarplexus.

3). Bridge the liver and spleen.

4). Then bridge the occiput with the tailbone.

5). Finally, you take the wrists of the person in each hand and balance the energy between them.

Allergies

These are usually caused by immunitary issues. To help allergies you want to bridge the thymus and the intestines.

Burns

Alleviating burns, can be done without putting a person into a mesmeric state.

1). Put both hands on both sides of the burn and focus the energy for about 3 minutes.

2). Ask them how they are and continue if needed.

Constipation

To help with constipation:

1). Use fascination.

2). Then do passes down the body.

3). Use Fascination as you gaze at intestinal area.

4). Use circular clockwise movements over the intestinal area without touching the stomach just using your energy, and continue doing this. (this clockwise circular movement causes digestion, both in the physical sense and in the emotional sense with bad emotions which we will talk about later.)

Eye Twitching

To help eye twitching place one hand over the forehead, and the other hand over the eye, you can switch as needed. Hold your hands in this position for 7 minutes or until normal.

Various Eye Problems

(For Someone Else)

Position your hands over the person's eyes and hold them there for 7 minutes or until normal.

(For Yourself)

Rub your hands together to warm them and make them tingle, then position your hands over your eyes, so that your palms are over your eyes, hold them there for about 7 minutes and do this about 3 times in a row. You can also hold your hands there until the warmth goes away and then rub them together again and reapply.

Kidney Stones

To help with kidney stones you can put your hands over the parathyroids on the sides of the throat, as this area controls the production of calcium in the blood, holding your hands here for a few seconds, and then bridge the kidneys and the area of the bladder by placing one hand over the kidney area from behind, and the other hand over the area above the bladder, from the front.

Loss Of Voice

To help bring back a lost voice, place both your hands over the sides of the voice box and keep them there for about 4 minutes everyday. This reduces inflammation and will help the person regain their voice.

Scrapes

This can be done without putting a person into a mesmeric state.

1). Focus your energy on the scrape for about 7 minutes per day until it is okay.

Back Issues

Discopathy

To help someone with discopathy:

1). Use Long passes down the back.

2). Bridge the occiput and the lower part of the back.

3). Make a triangular with your hands over the area where the pain is located.

4). If the body reacts, the treatment is working.

5). At the end, use long passes along the back to finish.

During the time you are working on the spine, you can use sound to help you. by using the EEEEEE and OHHHHHH sounds. This will cause the energy to regulate in the spin.

(To work on yourself)

Use the EEEE and OHHH sounds this will help you run energy up and down the spine. You can find these sounds in the advanced section.

Herniated Disks

To help someone with a herniated disk:

1). Use 2 or 3 long passes down the back.

2). Take both hands in triangular shape and aim them over the area where the pain is located until you feel it is time to move on.

3). Then move one of your hands away and close your other hand so all the fingers are together pointing out like birds beak and aim the energy at the kidneys.

4). Use 2 or 3 long passes at the end and balance the energy.

Sciatica

To help someone with sciatica:

1). Bridge the occiput, and the lower part of the back.

2). Then take both hands and make a triangle over the same place as the pain, and hold it there for a few seconds, or until you feel it's done.

3). If the body reacts, it means the treatment is working.

4). Then do 2 or 3 long passes along the back.

5). After that do 2 or 3 long passes along legs.

6). Finally do 2 or 3 long passes along the spine with hands in a butterfly movement.

The Endocrine System

To rebalance and help heal the endocrine system do the following:

1). Place one hand over the back of the head, and the other over the 3rd eye for a few seconds.

2). Bridge the forehead and the thyroid (throat).

3). Bridge the forehead and the stomach.

4). Bridge the forehead and the sexual organs.

5). Use the 3 sounds to regulate the energy (Ahhh: head, I: stomach, and O: belly).

6). End with 2 or 3 long passes from the head to the feet.

Knee And Joint Issues

To help someone with knee and joint issues:

1). Take both hands on both sides of the knee or joint and close your fingers together so the points of the 5 fingers point towards the knee in the beak shape, or you can use your 2 hands in the open palm style

2). Do circular rotations on the sides of the knee or joint.

Sexual Issues

These techniques below can help many different issues in this area.

For Women it can help with menstruation issues, fertility, low libido, infections, thrush, endometriosis, fibroids, cancers, libido and many others

For Men it can help with impotence, premature ejaculation, fertility, low libido, and many others. Generally when it comes to the sexual and urinary systems, the kidneys are the main source we need to heal.

General Sexual Balancing

To help a person generally balance their sexual energy:

1). Do 2 or 3 long passes, then aim your hands at the lower pubic region.

2). Put one hand over the forehead and one on the occipital lobe and balance holding your hands for a few seconds or until you feel it's time to move on.

3). Bridge the heart and abdomen.

4). Place one hand over the front of the body over the pubic region without touching and the other hand on the back over the tailbone area.

5). Then with your hands, bridge the kidney and adrenal area.

6). Finally do energisation on the ankles and then wake the subject up.

Menstrual Problems

To help someone with menstrual problems:

1). Place one hand over forehead area and the other over the occiput.

2). Do passes downward to solarplexus.

3). Bridge the forehead to the thyroid.

4). Bridge the forehead to the ovaries.

5). Bridge both kidneys.

Menstrual Problems Option 2

1). Bridge the forehead to the thyroid.

2). Bridge the forehead to the adrenal and kidney area.

3). Bridge the forehead to the pancreas.

4). Bridge the forehead to the genitals.

5). You can then focus more on the endocrine glands to help with the hormones. These areas are the pituitary, thyroid, parathyroid, thymus, and adrenal glands.

Erectile Dysfunction

To help someone with erectile dysfunction:

1). Bridge the forehead with the heart.

2). Bridge the forehead with the abdomen.

3). Bridge the occiput and the tailbone.

4). You can then focus more on the endocrine glands to help with the hormones. These areas are the pituitary, thyroid, parathyroid, thymus, and adrenal glands.

5). Do 2 or 3 long passes along the spine.

6). Do inverse pyramid with your two hands on the spine.

7). Do inverse pyramid on the kidneys and adrenals.

8). Do inverse pyramid on the spleen and liver.

9). Do regular pyramid at genitals.

Helping with Skin Diseases And Immunitary Issues

The technique below can help people heal that have skin and immunitary diseases such as Alopecia, worts, psoriasis, eczema, and lupus.

To Do:

Once the person is in a state, you then feel the left palm and feel the heat, then do the same with the right palm, if you feel one is colder than the other send energy into it, without touching it.

1). Go to the person's head put one hand in the front of the forehead and one in the back at the occiput to deepen the trance state.

2). Once you have held your hands here for a few moments you can move behind the person and put your hands over the top of their head. One hand over the right side of the brain, the other over the left side of the brain. As you do this the person will slip into a magnetic trance deeper and deeper

3). Make a bridge over the thymus and the solar plexus and stay there about 1 minutes, then move on to a bridge with the left hand over the liver and the right hand over the pancreas area. You will stay here for about a 1 minute.

4). Place your hand over the area of the skin with the problem and you will stay here for about 3 minutes.

5). Wake them up and ask them how that section of skin feels, if they feel a sensation there it means we have gotten results.

Dermatitis

Dermatitis is usually caused by immunitary issues. To help a person with this do a bridge with the thymus and the intestines.

Psoriasis

To help with psoriasis, focus on the liver, solar plexus, and Spleen. Do a circular motion with your hand over these three areas.

Psychosomatic Diseases

For psychosomatic problems, focus on the liver to help give relief for these.

Herpes

To help a person with herpes, you can focus your energy through your finger aimed at the affected area for atleast 3 minutes and ask them how they feel.

Magnetizing Water At The End Of A Session

You can magnetize water and use it at the end of a session. This increases the effects of the session. It should be given at the end of the session after the person has woken up and recovered. There are 2 methods to magnetize water.

Option 1

1). Do passes over the water for about 3-5 minutes this will allow the mesmeric fluid to fill the water and then when it is drunk it will heal from the inside as well.

Option 2

2). You can place a straw in the water and blow into the water. The mesmeric fluid in your breath will fill the water and energize it.

(Chapter 4) Emotional Problems, Phobias, And Addictions

Here we will learn how to heal mental traumas, emotional problems, addictions and phobias. Here again just by putting someone in the mesmeric sleep it will help them. The energy is intelligent and knows what to do, but with the techniques below you will be able to work much faster and heal much more effectively.

The Light Technique

This light technique at the end of various techniques below, solidifies the changes and makes things better and should be used at the end of a session, it should be 75 watts white light between 3-9ft or 1-3 meters distance, it can also be something like a candle as well which is what was used in the old days but the lower light can take longer to take effect.

To Use This Technique:

1). Have the person look at a light for about 30 seconds, no brighter than 75 watts, you don't need much, even a candle can work great.

2). Have them choose one word to express how they now feel after a treatment and have them say it out loud 3 times. For instance, free, liberated, etc. or they can just think about the word in their mind.

3). Then have them close their eyes and watch the outline of the light for about 30 seconds or until it fades into blackness.

4). Then have them open their eyes.

To Use This Technique To Get The Subconscious To Answer Questions For Us

Have the person look at the light and ask themselves a question they need their subconscious to answer. Then close their eyes and look at the traces of light and the answers should come to them.

TO ELIMINATE BAD EMOTIONS AND PROBLEMS

Arkeos Technique

To eliminate bad emotions and bring changes this technique works very well and is fairly easy. In addition it works fairly quickly. It works by affecting the energy of the body. So we ask them to choose an image that represents the emotion and then as we do clockwise circles over the solar plexus the image in their mind begins to change until it is completely different and they are free from the negativity of the emotion. This technique can also be done to yourself. If you are going to do it on yourself you will want to use the closure of the senses to put you in a state.

To Do Arkeos:

1). Ask the person if they know the emotion they have that they want to get rid of. It is not necessary for you as the mesmer to know the emotion, but they must.

2). Ask them what the emotion would look like if it had an image. The first thing that comes to mind and it is best if it's just an abstract image and not something real or complicated. Such as a shape like a circle or triangle. Oftentimes it can have a color as well, and that is fine.

3). Touch them in the solar plexus and tell them to imagine looking at the room through their solar plexus, to imagine how much wider the room would look to them.

4). Have them close their eyes and imagine the image they chose. But they must look at it from their solar plexus.

5). Do a few passes down to their solarplexus.

6). Then do a clockwise rotation over their solar plexus, this is the direction of digestion, you do this not by touching it but being close to the solar plexus as we do with passes, and tell them to continue to look at the image.

7). Continue to do rotations and keep your other hand behind them directly behind the solar plexus, then ask them if anything is changing. Eventually the image in their mind will begin to change. Continue on.

8). You can do downward frictions on the sides of their arms downward, then go to their knees and do downward frictions to the floor essentially moving the negative energy away from them. Then go back to the rotations on the solar plexus with the other hand behind. Then ask if things are changing.

9). You will continue to do this set until the image is completely changed.

10). Have them open their eyes and stare at the light, ask them if they had to choose 1 word to describe how they feel what would that be? Then have them say that word 3 times out loud as they look at the light and then close their eyes and view the outline of the light behind their eyes for about 20 or 30 seconds.

The Reduction To Nothing Technique

To work with a problem such as a person always being angry about something or they don't like, a cat at night or sounds in the next apartment or whatever.

1). First we use fascination.

2). Once the person is in fascination, you will basically ask them the same question over and over:

    a. "What is the worst of this problem?" When they answer you then ask,

    b. "And what is the worst of this (blank)?"

You will continue asking this questions going deeper and deeper into each answer until they are at a point where they don't know what to say. At this point then you will ask the final question.

3). "If you put that aside, what is left?": generally the answer will be something along the lines of "nothing" etc. It's the point of nothingness. The point where there is nothing left of the problem.

4). Then ask "What is the meaning of your problem now?" generally they will give you an answer of "It's not important" or "I feel better", etc.

5). After this, do the light technique: to block them in their current state where they are outside of their problem and no longer feel it's important.

PHOBIAS AND ADDICTIONS

Eliminate Phobias With The Sphere Of Light Technique

This technique eliminates phobias completely and works incredibly quickly.

1). Ask the person to remember the first time they had that fear or phobia.

2). Have the person look at a light for 20 seconds.

3). Have them close their eyes and look at their third eye as you lightly touch their third eye. Ask them to imagine the light continuing to go into their eyes and going to the back of their skull creating a Sphere of light.

4). You tell the person to continue to look at the third eye and while they are looking at their third eye, the sphere goes to the past event. It's important to let them know that they will not go to the event, they will stay here in the present, that only the sphere will go to the past. Tell them it's like a spiritual part of them going to visit the past event. Tell them when the sphere comes back, they will open their eyes and the phobia will be gone.

Important note: The person must not go to visit the past event, it's just the sphere that goes. If they go with the sphere they will not be relieved of the phobia. To explain it you can tell people that, the sphere goes and visits the past event but not us.

To Stop Smoking (OR Other Addictions) Using The Campanelli Method

This technique takes 90 seconds and works almost every time. It works very well, but first you must make sure they actually want to stop smoking. They have to want to be free from smoking for this to work.

1). First you ask them why they smoke, how long they have smoked, and why they want to quit. Ask them what their life would be like if they could quit.

2). (Optional)You can come behind them and shock them by putting a heavy hand on their shoulder then telling them something like "Today you will stop smoking" but you don't have to do this.

3). Once you have talked to them you tell them "This technique works 70% of the time, sometimes it works wonderfully, sometimes it doesn't work at all. We don't know why it works; it works because it works. Do you want to do it?" In reality it works almost every time but by saying this it changes their mind frame and keeps it from being a challenge if they can resist, to having them hope it works for them.

4). Then you tell them to close their eyes. Then you as the practitioner put one hand on the forehead and one on the occiput and gently rotate their head in a circle and say "let your mind be free".

5). Then while keeping the hand touching the forehead move the hand from the occiput to place it so it touches the center of the heart and make a bridge between the forehead and the heart hold this for about 30 seconds.

6). Then do friction passes from shoulders down the arms to the elbows, stopping at the elbows for a brief second, then continue with another friction pass from the elbows down to the forearms and to hands, stopping here for a brief second, and then continuing with the last friction pass from the wrists to the end of hands. This removes the energy.

7). Then go back and do a forehead and heart bridge for about 30 seconds.

8). Repeat the friction passes like before.

9). Then touch the forehead and place your other hand over the solar plexus without touching it holding here for about 30 seconds.

10). Repeat friction passes as before.

11). Tell them they can open their eyes, usually by this point they will have entered a state of trance.

12). Tell them for the next 48 hours they should focus on not doing their addiction and stay away from coffee, and alcohol.

(Chapter 5) Mesmeric Crises And Regressions

A crisis is a discharge of pent up hidden emotional energy. Traditional hypnosis talks about avoiding such things, but in reality, it should be embraced because It is very useful, and healing. When a person goes through a crisis, they are releasing all the negative pent up fear and trauma that is giving them issues in their daily lives whether physical illness, mental illness, or just blocking them from being happy. But it can be shocking the first time you see it and for bystanders as well. A person in crises can move, scream, or cry, or appear in great pain. Just remember the person is totally fine and in a state of peace inside even if they appear to be tortured outside. So you yourself must remain calm, because your energy will transfer to the client and to the observers as well. Stay calm and relax, the process will happen by itself, and you may have to let others, who are watching, know that it is completely normal and the person is okay, so they can feel calm too. If a bystander can not remain calm it is best you have them leave the room.

The emotional build up that is eventually released by a crisis, is caused by fear or traumatic events that never were discharged. Something that caused them to freeze or be in fear that they never recovered from. It could be public speaking or something more traumatic, that caused the emotional freeze, but the person never really shook it off. So when we cause a person to go into a crises, we are causing that person to feel that emotion but this time we cause them to move. This movement releases this pent up stuck energy and frees the person from all kinds of physical and emotional issues.

When working with a subject, sometimes a crisis can just come on, other times you have to find the emotion to work with to create the crises. If it does suddenly come on, just let it happen and follow the steps below. Every crisis is beneficial, the normal progression is that it starts out small, will peak sometimes loudly and intensely, and finally, no matter how intense, every crisis will end! So don't worry.

Some movements a person makes are symbolic, others are what they needed to do at that time when the emotion was first frozen in the person.

While a person can have a crisis while standing, it is better to put the person on the floor, when you are putting them into a crisis, because the floor will deepen the trance and allow them to move better. Once the crisis is at an end and things have calmed down you should play music to help regulate the body's energy.. An excellent choice is Moonlight sonata with glass harp, because the high and low pitches in the song. The high and low pitches move the energy up and down the spine to regulate the energy. We will talk more about sounds, and what sounds you need to use for what situation in the next chapter on advanced mesmerism.

The final thing to keep in mind is that you must wait until the person's crisis ends, and when they are in a positive frame before you wake them. Because, when you wake up a person in hypnosis, they will keep the state they had in trance, so you never want to wake them up when they are having a crisis and are in a negative state.

Crises can be increased by fascination and regression.

To Properly Work With A Crises

1st you must find the emotion.

2nd you must notice the movement of that emotion, (this is the movement the body wants to do because of the emotion). You can find this out by just watching the person and seeing what they are slightly moving.

3rd You must allow the movement and cause it to increase (The easiest way to do this is to create a state of quiet inside a person and then have them feel the emotion inside, before you start. Then encourage the movement once it starts until it becomes automatic.)

How To Work With A Person For Crisis

Step 1: Let the person speak about their problem and if possible, let the emotion show up. (You must find the emotion.)

You want to have the client speak about their problem, create a positive attitude, listen, be present, and have a quiet state of mind, this sends a subconscious message to the clients mind. As they talk they will begin to enter into their problem, and begin to feel the emotion. As you are listening start to gaze at the person

Step 2: Once they are done talking, do some kind of practical demonstration showing your competence, and that they are in good hands. This prepares them to let go and trust you.

For example:

You can use an eye blockage technique which we will explain below.

Or any number of little things to show your abilities.

<u>*Step 3:*</u> Frame the session.

Ask the person these 3 questions. If they really want to be free of their problem? Ask, how their life would be different without the problem? Are they ready to get rid of their problem now?

Once they say yes, they are ready and you can begin the process.

If you or they are unsure of the emotion that is causing the person to have problems you can use the following method before moving forward with the crises. This technique is also good for helping yourself as well.

The Eye Blockage Technique

Often people will have several emotions that affect them. But we can only work with one at a time. When you are working with a person and you and they are not sure which emotion is the most painful for them you can use this technique to find out. You can also use this on yourself as well.

1). Have the person close their eyes, with their eyes closed, have them look up at the top of their head for a few seconds, then still keeping their eyes closed bring their eyes back down where they would normally look. Tell them to not try to open or keep their eyes closed, just for them to see what happens.

2). Have them think of an emotion, then have them try to open their eyes and see if they open or want to stay closed. Stop thinking of that emotion and reclose your eyes

3). Have them think of a second emotion, then try to open their eyes again, have them stop thinking of that emotion and reclose their eyes

4). Finally have them think of a third emotion, then try to open their eyes again. Have them stop thinking of the third emotion and then close their eyes again.

5). When this is done, have them open their eyes and ask them which emotion caused them to want to keep their eyes closed. The stronger emotions normally cause you to want to keep your eyes closed.

6). When you know which emotion was the strongest and caused them to have trouble opening their eyes the most, that is the emotion you should work with first.

Once you have the emotion it is time to do the crises, and there are several methods to do a crises.

To Put Yourself In A Crisis, Or Place Someone In A Crisis Remotely

This can be done on yourself, or you can use it on someone else either in person or remotely

1). Have them close their eyes and feel in a state of quiet and relaxation, put them in trance by any of the methods we have discussed above. For yourself, you can use self fascination with the mirror followed by charges.

2). Have them find the emotion that caused them to have trouble opening their eyes, within them. Notice how their body changes. Do they breathe more, move an arm etc.? Have them increase this movement voluntarily. It will be voluntary at first, but then as things progress it will become automatic.

3). As they begin moving, encourage the movement even more. Tell them to move, you as the mesmer can encourage these movements by clapping rhythmically and also using the sound (Hah hah like a goose makes over and over,) Have them continue the movement until it starts to settle down a little. Make a bridge by putting a hand on the navel and another on the solar plexus, this helps to balance the energy.

4). (Once their movements slow down have them lay down.)

5). Tell them to Imagine there is a ball on their solar plexus, and that it is filled with this emotion. tell them to Kick it, have them put the right hand on the solar plexus, rotate it clockwise and have them tilt their heads left and right, and move and kick.)

6). After they settle down Play moonlight sonata for them.

7). When they open their eyes, they will feel a little better. Have them look at the light for about 20 seconds, then have them close their eyes and look at the trace of light on their closed eyelids. Have them look at it until the outline fades away.

Crises Method 2

This method is nearly identical but more for when you have the person infront of you and can touch and work on them physically.

1). Put them in a state and then talk to them, when you talk to them and once they start to show the emotion you can ask them to do something with their body. For example what do your hands want to do etc.

2). If they don't start to move, encourage them and you can even touch their arms to get them to do it. It is voluntary at that point, then it becomes automatic.

3). Once they start moving automatically you put them on the floor.

4). Then touch their solar plexus, this increases the bad emotion. While you touch the solar plexus you suggest that on the solar plexus there is a ball or a stone filled with the emotion that they are feeling, and they need to kick it, repeat this over and over until they begin to kick so it causes movement. This causes the beginning of the crises.

Sometimes it is not a big crisis so they start to kick and then stop and you are back to what appears to be square one. Just touch the solar plexus again, because touching the solar plexus causes the emotion to intensify and come out.

5). You can also tell them you are in a sea made of that emotion, put that emotion in your voice and the more emphasis the better you want to increase the emotion. Then you tell them to swim, or swim out of the emotion, or kick etc. The important thing is that they are moving. If they don't move their legs, touch their legs and encourage them to move them by saying swim, or kick, or move your legs.

6). After it is over you can play moonlight sonata.

7). Have them look at the light for about 20 seconds, then have them close their eyes and look at the trace of light on their closed eyelids. Look at it until the outline fades away.

Tips:

- If during a crisis the client starts talking saying things like "no" or "let me go" or anything, you must immediately stop the client from talking. Let them know they have to stop talking. They can make sounds if they want, but not talk. When they talk, it stops the emotion from creating physical movement, and in order for the crisis to liberate them they must have physical movement.

- If they are going through the motions but with no real anger or fear or emotion, tell them to stop and then suggest that the bad emotion is increasing and then have them start to swim or kick again. They need to be really in the emotion or the crisis won't liberate them either.

This is a regular more modern version of crisis. This is where we force the crises to come out by increasing the emotion, but now we are going to talk about the second type of crises which is an older technique and the one Mesmer used.

Mesmers Crisis Technique

This was Mesmer's method and personally my favorite as it's automatic. You can stimulate points of the body and if there is a need it will start the crises by itself. You don't need to start it like a regular crisis.

If there is no need for a crisis, then it doesn't start. It is a completely nonverbal technique.

Because of this, you can avoid regression in this approach, because you don't want to speak. With this technique, sometimes the crisis is big, and sometimes it's just something small, but it's automatic and will happen as much as the body and mind need so every reaction is good.

How To Do It:

Do the first 3 steps when initially working with the client as with a traditional crises but do not do regression or speak. If you spoke about their problem beforehand their subconscious is already directed towards helping with that problem.

You also don't need to bring out the emotion or increase it. Everything comes out automatically from the person's subconscious.

1). Do an initial induction and put them on the floor and do some more passes.

2). Do circular passes on both sides of the temples, to deepen their state. This is a very strong deepening technique.

3). Begin touching the hypnogenic points and using sounds, try using the sounds we talk about in the next chapter, for a few seconds to see which gives you a better reaction and then continue to use that one.

4). Start with grabbing both ankles at the same time and hold them for a few seconds to a minute or so, you will feel when it's time to move on. But generally it's about 30 seconds or so, while you do this you gaze at the person. Then slowly move up the body to the different hypnogenic or Farea points. The knees, then thighs, the belly, solar plexus, center of the chest, the shoulders, the temples, the third eye, and top of the head. Somewhere during the process it will start if it needs to.

5). Mix in random touches on the body to cause tension.

6). Once a reaction starts you can stop touching the hypnogenic points.

7). Do circular movements over the solar plexus. (Doing clockwise rotations over the stomach and solar plexus helps to let go of the emotion. You can also rotate over the liver in some cases as well.)

8). Do random noises with your hands near the person such as tapping on the floor, clicking your mouth, and snapping your fingers, etc.

9). When the person stops you can also play music like moonlight sonata. Afterward you can wake them up like normal, Use the light therapy as mentioned above, and have them take the time they need to come back.

10). Give them magnetized water at the end.

During any type of crisis, we are transforming the emotion into motion and this helps free the body. Afterwards they will feel liberated and healed. Sometimes they will feel tired, and it's important that afterwards you don't speak to them too much about the experience immediately after. You can ask them how they feel, and use the light therapy to solidify the results. Then after they recover and fully come back, you can ask them how the experience was for them.

How To Work With The Organs During Crises And To Relieve Blockages

All organs are related to an emotion. Each negative emotion affects a specific organ and the energy system it's connected to. Bad emotions are one of the worst things that cause energy blockages. These blockages can actually cause disease and damage to the corresponding organ, as well as the parts of the body connected to it energetically. We must understand which organ to work on when someone has a particular emotion. Knowing this allows us to do 2 things. First during a crisis we can work on the specific organ to increase the emotion which will allow for better healing. Second, when a person has an issue or disease in a particular organ and we find out they have had a lot of a certain emotion, we better know how to go about helping them.

The organs are part of energy centers in the body, and a problem in one energy center can cause problems in multiple other areas of the body. For example someone who has had a lot of sadness may develop lung blockages. These energy blockages could cause problems with the lungs but may also manifest as problems with the large intestine. So by knowing a person has had a lot of sadness and they are having problems with their large intestine it allows us to know that while we need to help with the large intestine we must also focus on the blockage in the lungs. We will explain this below. The important thing to remember is if there is a sickness or disease relating to an energy system you want to focus on eliminating the negative emotion and curing the main organ as well as working on the organ showing symptoms.

Going back to our lung example. If someone is having a lot of problems with their large intestine and you find they have had a lot of sadness. We want to remove the negative emotion, and work on the large intestine, but also on the lung area as well. Because this is the source of the blockage, and that will help reduce the problems in the rest of that energy system. If not, you may eliminate one problem, but another may pop up. Remember, it is the emotion and energy blockage to the organ that are the cause, the rest are symptoms. Eliminate the cause and the symptoms go away.

Also, while we are talking about mesmeric crisis here, remember that this holds true even if we are not using the crisis. For example we could eliminate the emotion with Arkeos, then induce trance and do passes and begin to unblock the organs and the energy centers, without going into crisis. However, crisis is a great tool for eliminating the stuck trauma and locked emotions of the past, so it is recommended.

During a crisis, you can work with magnetic passes on specific organs to bring the emotion out that corresponds to that organ. Normally we want to increase the emotion before a crisis, because the more the emotion is out when we start a crisis the better it will be. In addition to passes you can also touch those areas of the body to bring the emotions out. You can also use your finger to point to and gaze at the corresponding organ. Even when a person's eyes are closed the gaze still works because the subconscious mind feels it.

The Liver - It is related to anger and frustration. Anger causes blockages in the liver and causes problems in other parts of the body. The liver system can affect the liver, gallbladder, fingernails and eyes. Blockages in the liver can show up as problems in any of the connected systems listed above, including digestion problems, addictive behaviors, and eye sight problems. Many eye problems are not due to getting old but are related to blockages in liver energy and by working on removing the blockages and helping the liver many times eyesight problems will heal on their own. In severe cases blockages in this system can lead to heart attack or strokes. So, if you are working on someone with the emotion of anger or frustration, you can work on the liver before or during the crises to bring the anger out. You can cause the emotion to grow by stimulating the liver before going into crises, and then work on helping it and any affected organ after. When we work on helping the liver we must also work on the gallbladder too, because they are so connected. Also remember that the opposite emotion that damages an energy center can help unblock it. In the case of the liver, happiness will help it.

The Stomach and Pancreas - This is related to anxiety and worries. Oftentimes people that think too much for work, or just worry in general, will get blockages here. The stomach system can affect the stomach, pancreas, lips, and spleen. Blockages in this system can show up as digestive problems, symptoms of arthritis, tightness or other issues with the neck and shoulders, or even contribute to diabetes. So, we can use magnetic techniques on this area after a crisis. Often you will want to do clockwise circles over the stomach area; this helps to digest the bad emotions that have caused the crises, and will help to allow the person to let go of the emotions. With the stomach the emotion of peace will help it.

The Lungs - Related to sadness and depression. Sadness and depression damages the lungs and its energy system which includes the lungs, sinuses, nose, throat, large intestines, hair, skin, and teeth. So blockages can show up as any of these areas being affected or having problems. So, if a person you are working with has sadness, you can start with passes and then spend more time on the lungs. Then you can use circular passes. You want to increase the emotion so do it clockwise.

The Heart - This is related to hate. So when a person has this emotion, this is the organ we need to work on. Hate causes disease and issues in the heart, tongue, and small intestines. We can work on it in a similar way as above. However with the heart it's important to note that we don't want to point at it with our fingers. We only want to use our palms. The energy from our palms is more inline with the heart energy. The energy from our fingers is different from the heart energy. It won't physically hurt the person but it's not good for healing. Finally the emotion that helps the heart the most is gratitude. So having the person feeling gratitude for what they have will also work wonders here.

The Kidneys - This is related to fear. Fear damages the kidney energy and kidney energy is life force energy, and one of the most important energy points in the body. The kidney system includes the kidneys, ears, hair, and reproductive organs, including women's breasts. Blockages can show up in any of these areas, or even with a feeling of reduction of strength, loss of stamina, gaining weight or having hearing problems, etc.

REGRESSIONS

Regressions are very easy. In mesmerism we work on states not on words, so the words you use are not that important. You can do these regressions with yourself, with a person remotely over the phone, internet, or in person. Regressions can be used to bring a person back to any point in time they had a trauma, want to remember something, or just let something negative go.

Most trauma happens because a piece of the person gets locked into the time when the trauma happened, but now that it's over they can not do anything about it. By doing a regression the person can go back to that time and now since it is fresh and current to them they can begin to react and release the trauma before it becomes locked in them again. Because of this, often we will do a regression first before going into a crisis, but it's not always necessary.

Note: When we have someone jump into different parts of their past, we can use the sounds AAA RAAM. The RAAM is forcefully said as it's pushed out. Ram traditionally is connected to power and fire and so it will clear the path when the person arrives, so if they are going somewhere bad in their past, they will arrive in power. It's like they are burning away the problem as they arrive. This allows them to do a regression easier.

When you do self-regression, you don't want to say AAA RAAM too many times, so if you are not getting results, go back and do more charges.

If a person feels cold after they complete a regression that is a good sign it means the parasympathetic system was activated and they were in a good state of relaxation

To Do A Self Regression Or To Work With Someone Remotely

This first method can be done anywhere, but it also works great for remote work, and for self-regression. An interesting side note is that a variation of the technique below is said to, in the past, have been able to give the practitioner the ability to self project their essence to another place so that they could speak to a person far away. However that is a very old application and we will not be focusing on that here. In the case below you will use a mirror for fascination and move your hand in a counter clockwise circle so you can see.

To Do A Regression:

You may do passes if you are with a client in person or do Charges if you are working on yourself or a client remotely, where doing traditional passes would be difficult or impossible.

After the 3rd cycle of passes or charges, have the subject inhale, and bring their attention to their heart, while having them imagine hearing a sound like a high pitched E.

Inhale and then tell them with that sound and with their eyes open to go back to a moment in their past as you the mesmer says RAAM to ensure the way is safe for them.

Then from that point if you wish, you can have them leave that time and go into another moment, as you the mesmer says AAA RAAM. You may repeat this as many times as you wish. However once you at the point you want them to be in the past

Then you tell the person to look at you, as you take your hand and move it counter clockwise in a circle infront of them, as if creating a tunnel or vortex.

Tell them to answer mentally, or you can ask them to answer outloud to these questions as you continue to move your hand circularly counter clockwise.

1). Are you alone or with someone?

2). Is it Day or night?

3). Are you standing or moving?

4). After they tell you more you can say something along the lines of "Now you decide to take control and to be back in power again". Have them Inhale and feel their feet in the situation in the past, then have them exhale.

5). Continue through another round of charges, or passes, then continue to the next step.

6). Then you say something like "Now you feel complete, it's just you, it's as if you have taken back control." You can also tell them that they can go back and do it again if they feel they still have some part of them back there."

7). Do another round of charges or passes again.

8). Then say something like "And now you are here in the present, when I count to 3 you will close your eyes, 123 close your eyes", pause for a second or 2, then say, "now open your eyes."

9). Now have them look at the light and do the light technique.

How To Do A Regression Going Into A Crises

To begin with, to work with a client, ask them these questions to create pain so they want to change their situation. You may word them how you wish but these are the questions you need to get answers to.

1). How many times has this problem stopped you in your life?

2). How would your life be different if you didn't have this problem?

3). Do you want to eliminate this problem?

These 3 questions enhance motivation, you need motivation to help a person heal from these emotions. They must want to be free, otherwise there is no point in moving forward.

Regression To Help Eliminate A Past Trauma

1). Ask them the 3 important questions above.

2). Have them touch the part of the body where they feel the emotion is stored or held in their body.

3). Once they feel the emotion, do an induction.

4). You can say something like "On the count of three you will go back to the very first time you ever felt this emotion, look into my eyes, 3..2...1 you are back, it's the very first time you felt this emotion. Where are you? Are you alone or with someone?" If they hesitate or seem to think, tell them to say the first thing that comes to their mind, where are they?

5). Then you ask them more questions, what is around them, how old are they, etc. This deepens the regression.

6). Then you can use different therapies to calm the person either working on their solar plexus or doing crises.

To create the crises from this point you can ask them, What movement does your body want to do, or what do you want to do with your hands etc., When they give you an answer encourage it by telling them to move. Then encourage them to move again and again stronger and stronger. As you, the mesmer, breathe heavily out loud as you do this, and this will encourage the crisis to start.

7). You can also clap rhythmically to encourage the crises to come out further, as you encourage them to move.

8). You must wait until the crisis ends, and not wake them up too early or they will keep the negative state they were in.

9). At the end, play music to regulate their energy, and then wake them and have them look at the light and use the light technique.

How To Do A Free Regression So They Can Go Forward Or Back In Time

You can use a Free Regression where we do not tell the subject where to go. This can be useful if they need to go to the future as well, and see what their life could be like, this is useful for people looking for a path in life.

1). Put them in trance.

2). Ask them to look for a light and when they find it they can move their finger to tell you.

3). When they find the light tell them to go to it, and go into another place and another time.

4). Then you may ask them where they are, when they are, etc. from here you may begin to ask them questions

5). Afterwards, put them on the floor and give them time to deepen their state.

6). Then you can continue with magnetic passes, and finally wake them.

How To Do A Past Life Regression

This can be useful if someone has a trauma from a past life.

1). Do an induction.

2). Tell them to continue to look at you, as you do counter clockwise circles as if creating a tunnel or vortex. Tell them you will count from 3-1 and then at 1 they will go to a moment in their past.

3). Move your hand in counter clockwise circles in front of them and say 3 2 1 you are in the past. Then you may ask questions such as Where are you, are you alone or with somebody? Ask them if it's day or night? If they seem to hesitate or need to think, tell them to answer quickly. Tell them to Look at you, then ask them questions like what's their name? and etc.

4). After you get a general idea of where and when they are, you can then say that you will count from 3-1 and on 1 they will be at the very last moments of the person's life. You can then count 321 and say, Now we are now at the last moment of the person's life. Ask them if they can see what's happening? Remember again the exact wording is unimportant, as long as it's similar you will be fine.

5). Then you can say that you will count from 3-1 and on 1 we will go to the most significant part of his life 321, how old is he. It is important to separate the past life from the person, so we dont say how old are you, in a past life regression, always say how old is he or she, this will help keep the 2 personalities separate. You can then ask what is happening? If they are having trouble seeing anything, ask them if they can widen their gaze and see. Ask them, what movement does (he or she person from last life) want to do? Then whatever movement it is, encourage them to do it again and again. This causes the regression to go into a crisis. From here you just follow the steps for a normal crisis.

6). Bring them back to the present as before, so something like I will count from 3-1 and on 1 you will be back in the present in this life. 3,2,1 you are back in the present, back in this life, then when you are sure they are back, wake them up.

Calming Techniques

If someone is in a regression and starts to get too scared or emotional there are a couple techniques you can use to calm them and help them resolve their conflicts.

The Focusing on 2 Things Technique

This technique works great with fascination it works on the principle that if we bring the subject in the present to feel TWO THINGS (breathing and looking at you) he will no longer be able to focus on the emotion.

Using this technique is very simple:

1). Say: "Look at me now and feel your breathing."

2). "Can you feel the emotion? They should say no, and should be okay at this point.

Focusing on an External Element Technique

This technique works on the principle of bringing the person's attention to an external element, by doing this we will change their attention and weaken the emotion.

To Do:

1). Say: "Widen your gaze and see if there is something that calms you."

2). Then watch and notice that they calm down

Going to the Point of Birth Technique

If we bring the person to the point of birth, their problems do not exist yet and they will be able to feel a positive feeling

1). Tell the person in crisis to go to the moment of birth and look inside yourself. Do you see a point of light? If they say yes, that is good and have them just relax.

Going to the point of Death Technique

This technique is only for past life regressions. Like the technique above if we go to the point of death where the person is dead in the past life they no longer have any problems and will be able to feel a positive feeling at this point.

1). Go to the moment of death, and look inside yourself. Do you see a point of light?

Generally they shouldn't and just see nothing and this will bring them into a calmness.

As with all of the techniques above, you will notice a shift in the person, either a marked calmness or, often once the person has been calmed you will hear them breath out and their body may go limp, this is a great sign that they are calm and the issue has been resolved, you can let them rest for a moment then bring them back to the present and out of trance.

(Chapter 6) Advanced Techniques

Advanced Exercise

This next exercise will create new neural connections and connect the two hemispheres of your brain, this will allow you to increase your abilities.

Hot And Cold Water Technique

1). Fill 2 bowls one with hot water and one with cold water.

2). Place your left hand in the hot water and your right hand in the cold water.

3). Try to feel as though the hot water is the cold water and the cold water is the hot water. It will take some time but by doing this you will create new neural pathways that will increase your magnetic abilities.

Using Mesmerism To Mesmerise Through Solid Walls

Mesmerism is energy and energy has no distance and no obstacles. Because of this we can use mesmeric passes and mesmerize someone on the other side of a wall. You will need to practice this until you get it down, so just have someone stand on the other side of a wall and begin to do passes, feel presence, and the connection with the person, and have fun.

USING SOUNDS TO CREATE MESMERIC TRANCE AND TO HEAL

Using Sounds

Sounds can be used for self healing as well as healing others, because when we work on ourselves it can be difficult to do passes on ourselves, sounds are a good option. When working on yourself you can make the sounds or once you have more experience, simply make the sound in your mind. The sound in your mind will still cause the energy to move.

These sounds, when made, can also be used to entrance others all by themselves and can be used for distance healing such as through zoom or on the phone when we wouldn't be using in person passes. The sounds are very ancient, and are useful since they block the mind. It is said that the sirens of ancient Greece used sounds to fascinate and lure sailors to their doom and stories have been told of fascinators in old days using sounds to heal, entrance, and even cause crops to grow. The sounds below can only be used to heal, and when added to your techniques can be a vital ally.

__SH__ sound - (pronounced SHHH) -

Occult properties: It is the sound of fire, It's color is red, it is hot, and warming.

__M__ sound - (pronounced Muuh) -

Occult Properties: it is the sound of water, It's color is blue marine, It is cold, and cooling.

Normally you can heal a lot with the SH, and M sounds because they are hot and cold. These 2 sounds can be used on almost every part of the body. Use the sounds like you would a regular hot or cold pack. If there is inflammation you want to use the M sound to cool. M is useful and can help heal a lot of different problems including neuromuscular problems.

__AE__ sound - (pronounced like deep Uuuuh) -

Occult Properties: It is the sound of earth, its color is brown, It signifies heaviness.

This sound can be used rarely in situations for headache too.

Sounds To Balance Energy And To Entrance

**E** sound - (pronounced like a high EEEE) -

Occult properties: It is the sound of air, its color is light blue, it signifies lightness.

This sound can be used for headaches, it also brings the energy up to the head.

**O** sound - (Pronounced like a deep OHHHH) -

This can be used to bring the energy to the root, or tailbone at the base of the spine. Which is a vital energy point. It strengthens the kidney energy, and can help balance the energy in the body. It can also be used for healing sickness, and in some countries monks will form a circle around a sick person and just say O until the person heals.

**Ah** sound - (pronounced AHHHH) - can be used to bring energy to the chest and heart.

You can use the O, E, Ah sounds in combination and in order as passes to cause the person to go into trance. This causes the energy to be moved by the sound from the tailbone up the spine to the head and back to the chest and heart area. This balances the energy which is useful for healing. This again is useful if you can't do passes, for example if you are working over the phone or for distance work through ZOOM etc, but can also be used in conjunction with passes if you want.

To use sounds you must try them for about 2-5 seconds and then see if a person is better or worse. If they are better, continue, with the same sound. If they are worse, switch to another sound and try that. Until you find the sound that improves them.

Putting Sounds Into Water

Sound is vibration, and energy, and so it makes sense that this vibration and energy can be used to affect the things around it. Water is a strange substance that we are only beginning to understand, but it has memory and can actually be transformed by thoughts and intentions on a quantum level. This makes water very powerful and there are some very useful things we can do with it. We can use sound to change the quality of water and use that water to help heal or eliminate pain.

When using sounds with water we normally use only the sh and Muh sounds. In addition You can put an idea in water with intention, allowing you to use the water as a type of influence or hypnotic carrier. When you use the sounds to magnetize water, you want to send them through a living subject, as this amplifies the vibration.

To Use Sounds With Water

1). Have the person hold the glass of water and make the Shhh sound for about 5 seconds the vibration will go through the water.

2). Then have them try the water after and see if it makes them feel better.

3). Then make the Muh sound, and have the vibration go through the water. Then have them try the water after and see if it makes them feel better.

4). Ask the person if they feel a difference in the ridge of the palm of the hand between 2 sounds.

You want them to feel a difference, but it doesn't matter what. The ridge will feel the vibration and energy more than the rest of the hand because it is more sensitive energetically.

5). Whichever sound makes them feel better is the one you will use to finish off charging the water. Then have them finish drinking it, and it will help their condition.

Placing Spoken And Unspoken Commands Into The Water

With water, You can also put spoken and unspoken commands into the water. It is an intention being put into the water, and this can also give physical and mental effects. This water will increase the effects of a magnetic session.

Placing Ideas Into Water

You can also put an idea into the water. Imagine the idea inside the water and that you see it in the water like you were looking into a crystal ball. Then drink the water. To do this you must put the person into a hypnotic state first then have them imagine the idea in the water and then drink it to get the results.

ECSTASY

The state of ecstasy is very important, and the basis for doing more advanced techniques. There are different levels of ecstasy. When we go into ecstasy we go to the source. It causes the energy to rise up through our spine and go into the pineal gland in the brain, which is incredible for healing, and causes a feeling of ecstasy which is where this technique gets its name from. You can use it even in a normal session, as It's easy to do. Normally when people go into ecstasy their heads go back, also in many cases you can see their hands raise from their sides, like they are levitating, and they tend to go into a cataleptic state, especially when it's done in front of a mirror.

When you are putting someone in ecstasy it's very important to stimulate the third eye point and the top of the head, where the crown chakra is. In the self exercise below we stimulate these points when we begin to inhale from the eyes and exhale from the top of the head. When you are working on someone else you can even stimulate the back of the spin as this is where the energy flows through to reach the pineal gland. When a person goes through ecstasy and comes back they are not the same, they feel different, and this is because they have had connection with the source.

While you can go straight into Ecstasy, When you want a stronger ecstasy, put the person into somnambulism first. Once in ecstasy you can ask the person questions and they will answer with more clarity, and you can also attract them by using the pull techniques as well as others and they will follow. Sometimes they may even begin to dance.

Self Exercise And Remote Technique

You can use this technique for yourself or use it to put someone else in ecstasy remotely.

Sit down, and look at a light infront of you for about 30 seconds and then close your eyes, and look at the outline of the light shining in your closed eyes. Inhale, hold your breath and bring your awareness to your feet. Exhale, then inhale, holding your breath, and feel the sensation of your legs, exhale, inhale, holding your breath and feel your torso, exhale, and inhale, holding your breath and feel the sensation of your neck and arms, exhale, inhale and hold it as you notice the awareness of your head. Exhale, and repeat the process again to your head.

Then after that, you inhale and imagine you're inhaling from the feet and exhaling from the top of the head. Then imagine you are inhaling from the navel and exhaling through the top of your head, then inhale from the heart and imagine you exhale from the top of the head. Inhale from the eyes and exhale from the top of the head. Continue inhaling from your eyes and exhaling from the top of your head. Every memory, and image you have just let it go out the top of your head.

(Play moonlight sonata on glass harp.)

This will cause you or the subject to go into ecstasy.

To come back

Slowly inhale and have the air enter from the heart and go out from the top of the head

Then inhale again and have the air enter from the belly and then go out from the top of the head, then inhale and have the air enter from the feet and go out from the top of the head. Open your eyes. Then suddenly say STOP, tell yourself or the person to feel their body, feel the weight of their body, tell them to see everything, then tell them to hear everything.

You always must reintegrate yourself. So if you STOP immediately after you do ecstasy and reconnect with your senses it will help a person come back. If you don't, they will stay in a dreamy state and not be able to fully come back 100%.

To Put Someone Into Ecstasy

1). You can use the eye blockage technique first as this helps the process but you don't need to.

2). Do fascination first - this increases the ability to get them into ecstasy.

3). Close their eyes.

4). Do passes towards the solar plexus.

5). Leave the one hand behind the head and the other go down to the solar plexus.

You are watching to see when their head goes back as this is the sign they are going into ecstasy. You can help this process by just slightly pushing or pulling the shoulder back, it will cause the head to adjust.

6). Put one hand in back and one hand infront of solarplexus as we need to work with somnambulism first. So just keep the hands there until they start to go into somnambulism.

7). Then go in front of the person and take your left hand from the left side across the chest towards their right lower side. These are cross passes, then do right hand from the right shoulder and across the side to the lower left side.

8). Then go behind and do backward passes with both hands, pulling the essence from the third eye to the top of the head or, from the top of the head to the sky like you are straightening hair above the head, or you can do a combination of both techniques if you like.

9). Make the EEEE sound to make the energy rise.

You want to watch for the person's head to rise and go back; this is the specific sign of ecstasy. You can also play music to help the process or just keep using the EEEE sound.

10). Put one hand on the occiput and the other on the tailbone. This increases ecstasy. In addition, using the palm of your hand or your fingers to tap the third eye can stimulate the point and help the person go in deeper.

Another sign that people that are going into ecstasy do, is they raise their arms up from their sides.

Tip: You can also increase and speed up the process of putting someone into ecstasy with this simple technique.

Once the person has reached catalepsy, place the person's arms in a prayer position or open receptive as people who praise God in church often do, this actually helps cause the energy to rise to the pituitary, and increases the effects. While Ecstasy is good to do, it can create an addiction to the state if done often.

Waking Someone From Ecstasy

The process of bringing someone out of ecstasy is a little different than our other techniques. It is necessary to reintegrate the subject when waking them up from ecstasy. If you just wake them up directly, they will wake up, but be out of it, but in this state you can then put them back into somnambulism very quickly and easily.

To Wake Them Up

1). You first must do downward passes.

2). Then put your thumb on their third eye and your fingers on their head. They slowly lower their heads. This speeds up the process of waking them up.

3). Then you just do upward passes, fan their face or blow on them.

4). Once they come to. Stay STOP Then tell them to hear what's around them... see what's around them... feel their body.

This allows them to reintegrate into the present world.

And that's it.

ADVANCED SOMNAMBULISM

This is a deeper, more advanced level of somnambulism and can be used for more advanced techniques. Again as mentioned above we can use Somnambulism and this technique to get more psychic phenomenon. Such as having a person be able to find lost items, or knowing which items are hidden in a room and where they are etc. We get this type of somnambulism by stacking inductions one on top of the other. This causes a deeper somnambulism that you could not normally get from just one simple induction. When using this technique you want to encourage the person to move as this increases the trance.

To Put Someone In Advanced Somnambulism

1). Put them in ecstasy first then wake them suddenly.

2). Then close their eyes and make sounds on the left and right sides of the head by the ears, and around her head. One of the easiest ways to do this is by snapping your fingers around their head and on both sides of their ears.

3). By now you are probably seeing some movement such as their hands moving strangely. Ask them what their hands are doing and encourage them to continue the movement.

4). Make more sounds, and they will continue to move more, and go deeper.

5). When done wake as normal.

MAGNETIC BALANCING

This technique is very similar to energisation but can be used on yourself or others remotely. It's very refreshing and increases your energy. It balances energy similar to a bridge. But it's much easier to use on yourself. So while you can use it on someone else, you can also use it to help heal yourself when you feel like you might be getting sick.

To Magnetically Balance Yourself And Others Remotely

1). Put feet on the floor, and close your eyes.

2). Begin to breath and As you breath feel your right and left feet at the same time, then exhale.

3). Inhale, feel both legs at the same time then exhale.

4). Inhale and feel the lower part of the torso, both the right and left part.

5). Inhale and feel the upper part of the torso, both the right and left side, exhale.

6). Inhale and feel both arms at the same time, exhale.

7). Inhale, feel the neck and face, both right side and left side together and exhale.

8). Inhale ,feel both legs at the same time, exhale.

9). Inhale and feel the front and back of the lower torso at the same time.

10). Inhale and feel the front and back of the upper torso at the same time, exhale.

11). Inhale, feel the front and back of the head,, exhale.

12). Inhale, feel the right and left, front and back of the feet, exhale.

13). Inhale, feel both legs, right and left, front and back, exhale.

14). Inhale, feel the front and back, left and right of the lower torso, exhale.

15). Inhale, feel the upper torso, front and back , right and left, exhale.

16). Inhale and bring awareness to your stomach, close the pelvis muscles, and exhale.

17). Then on the count of 3 open your eyes. 1, 2, 3, open your eyes.

Magnetic Circle For Group And Long Distance Healing

When you do a circle with a group of people, magnetism can be increased. It can even be used to heal remotely even if they don't know the person they can imagine the person in the center and it will help heal them.

To Do:

1). Have the people that wish to experience it or be healed to stand in the center of the circle

2). Have the others, that are assisting make a circle around the people in the center. We want to have more people outside the circle than are in the circle.

3). The people in the circle will close their eyes and just relax and do nothing.

4). The people outside the circle first will join hands.

5). Tell them to feel the energy going from around the circle going through their left arm through them and out their right arm into the person's arm next to them.

6). You as the practitioner make the sounds OOOO EEEEE AAAA.

7). Have the people outside the circle stop, and open their eyes and begin doing passes towards the people in the center. This will begin to affect the people in the center. Then you as the practitioner can take the people in the center to the ground and work on them from there.

8). When you are done just wake the people in the center up like you normally would.

Magnetic Circle Version 2

This version will magnetize the people who are making the circle allowing you to heal a larger group just by yourself.

1). Have everyone stand in circle.

2). You as the practitioner need to feel your body and stay present.

3). Have them Imagine bringing their heart into the center of the circle.

4). Have them Imagine at this point they also bring the heart of the other people into the center as well.

5). Now have them imagine an energy that goes around the circle, going into their right arm and through them and then out their left arm and into the persons arm next to them.

6). Use the sounds OOOO EEEEE AAAA.

7). You as the practitioner must always be present and feel your body to keep from going into trance.

8). You can then leave the circle but connect the hands of the people together so the chain is not broken.

9). Begin working on them and taking them to the ground as they are ready.

10). Wake them up as normal when done.

The 10 Energy Plexus Technique

This can be used for pain or even energy balancing whether people are sitting or laying. It can also be used after a crisis to balance their energies. There are 10 energy points that are like energy lines that run horizontally across the human body.

To help eliminate a pain, you simply take the energy plexus right above the point of pain, and grab the energy bar imagining you are really pulling something out away from the body and bring it down to the level with the pain and push it in place.

Then grab that bar and pull it out imagining you are really pulling out the pain and bring down to the next plexus point level and push in place until you have gone through all the plexus to the feet. Then you take the bar from the feet, pull it out and bring it to the ground. You do this as if you are connecting the bars together.

Then do some long passes and then you wake the person up and say something positive like feel better now? Never ask if the pain is gone or where the pain is now, because they will start to search to see if they can feel the pain and could bring the pain back. By saying feel better now, they don't search for the pain so it's a much more positive way of asking.

If the pain is located in the head we need to use other techniques because there is no plexus above the head to start with.

The energy plexus bars are located:

1). At the crown chakra.

2). The 3rd eye.

3). The jaw line.

4). The arms plexus located right at the top of shoulders and the middle of the back. This is the area used to pull people back when we do magnetic attraction pulls.

5). The heart level.

6). The solar plexus level.

7). The navel (you can hit this point to get energy).

8). The genital area.

9). The knees.

10). The feet (the contact with the earth).

Clairvoyance

You can use mesmerism to cause clairvoyance and make people see things in water, fire, or in a mirror. It can be people, places, or accessing your intuition for answers to questions.

Note: Using reflected light increases clairvoyance. The light of the moon can be very useful. In nature, like in a Forest or park etc, the moon reflected on a lake or river is very strong and can actually be too strong in some cases. But you can even do clairvoyance inside a home.

Warning: You must use presence when doing clairvoyance. You can use clairvoyance to see and get ideas, but afterwards you must always bring those ideas back with you and get back to present. Or you risk being lost to viewing only visions.

There are several steps with the process:

1). Have the person concentrate on what they want to see for about 30-60 seconds before you begin because this tells the subconscious what you want to view.

2). Put them in a state.

3). They will begin to see something.

4). Have them acknowledge what they see by telling you out loud and this will encourage more and clearer visions.

Clairvoyance By Gazing Into Pools Of Water

You should have good nutrition and eat healthy as bad nutrition can cause you to not see things well, or have bad visions. Also where you work affects things as well. Working at night increases your vision, and in conjunction with being in nature like at a lake is even stronger.

When doing this method a person will normally begin to see a mist in the water. They must look into this mist and concentrate on it and it will allow them to see.

Things Needed

Take a clear round glass or crystal bottle or bowl of water (It must be round) and have the person viewing the bowl directly Infront of them at the height of their eyes so they can look directly into the bowl. A variation is to have the person look at the water from above.

Have the background behind the bowl a neutral color, you can place a white paper or black paper or just have a uniform color of paint.

Have a reflected light, not too strong, and not directly shining on the water. It could be a light or even 2 candles on both sides of the crystal bowl.

You can also take a piece of paper and have the person draw a small picture of what the person wants to see. Then put it under the bowl. This guides and suggests to the mind what vision you want

Steps With Induction

1). Have the person stand and use fascination on them it works very well for this technique, but it is not necessary you can start with them viewing the bowl directly.

2). Wake them up, then close their eyes.

3). Do some downward passes and then stay on the solarplexus, this will develop somnambulism. Then have the person open their eyes and look into the bowl.

4). Go behind the person, and Put your 2 hands above both hemispheres of the brain without touching. One hand on the left top of the head and the other on the right top of the head.

5). Ask 2 important questions that must be answered yes 1. Do you want to see? 2. Will you allow the Universe to let you see?

6). Stay with your hands in their place for a few seconds, it is important to keep your hands here as it will speed up the results much more.

7). Ask if they see a mist inside the water, if yes, have them look inside the mist.

8). You can do some downward passes on the sides of the head and then you can ask them to describe what they see if they are seeing anything. If they are, have the person tell you what they are seeing as this will encourage more visions. Make sure to keep them talking.

9). Once you are at this point you can just keep your hands in place above the head. Make sure not to ask for precise details but just have them tell you what they see, because if you ask for too much precision it risks ruining the visions, and invoking the imagination. They will begin to actually feel things too such as temperature etc.

10). It is not good to just stop the vision so you must ask the person if they want to stop. Once they say yes, you can bring them back out.

To Bring Them Back Out

1). Move your hands from the top of their head and then balance them with a forehead and solar plexus bridge for about 20-30 seconds.

2). Downward passes on the front and back of the person to the solarplexus.

3). Upward passes to bring the person back, or you can tap the side of their face, etc..

4). Once they are awake, have them look at the light so their unconscious can process the information for about 20-30 seconds.

5). Have them close their eyes and then you need to cover their eyes with one hand and place the other hand over their occiput. While they view the traces of light.

6). Blow on the persons face to open the eyes.

7). Do Fenix Method.

Steps Without Induction

1). Have the person sit in the seat facing the bowl of water.

2). Go behind the person, and   put your hands over their eyes to close the eyes.

3). Face away from them, with your back to them, and move an imaginary sword in a circle.

4). Move to all fours sides again facing away from them as you move the imaginary sword in a circle.

5). Open their eyes, then have the person look at the bowl as you place your hands above the 2 hemispheres of the brain.

6). Have them tell you what they see.

7). Side passes down the head and the arms, then put the hands back in the original position above the head.

8). Have the person continue to tell you more.

Steps To Wake Them Up

1). Remove your hands from the top of their head, balance them with a forehead and solar plexus bridge for about 20-30 seconds.

2). Do upward passes or tap on the face to wake up.

The Fenix Method To Finalize The Process

You can have them take the images they saw, close their eyes, put their hand on their belly and then imagine burning the images and having the burned images going up their spine and out their head. This helps the mind to reconstruct everything and make the ideas better. Always burn the ideas, they will reconstruct in the mind better after, always.

Using The Cagliostro Method For Yourself Alone

This technique was created by Count Alessandro Cagliostro who was a magician, alchemist, mesmer and free mason. I would encourage you to look deeper into this man, and his life.

You can use this technique to view things by yourself but it can take a little longer and the technique is a little different

1). Move in a square and go to all fours sides facing away from the center of the square as you move an imaginary sword in a circle.

2). Go infront of the bowl.

3). Put your hands ontop of both hemispheres of the brain just like above.

4). View inside the bowl of water and when you see the mist, start to either speak outloud or think by describing what you see. The more you speak the more you will see and enter into a trance.

5). At a certain point the vision will finish or you will feel like closing your eyes. Then close your eyes and stay quiet.

6). Afterwards look at the light, close your eyes, and imagine you are burning the images and they are traveling up your spine. Then you can open your eyes.

Magic Mirrors

You can use the mirror to have visions in as well, you will not see as much as the Cagliostro water method but it will give you the answers you seek. You can use this to find out what someone is doing, or what is happening somewhere else, or what you will do in the future, or something in the future. There should be a person in the question of what you want to know.

How To Do:

1). Go infront of a mirror and have a strong light reflected in it.

2). 1st decide what you want to know, what question you want answered.

3). Go infront of the mirror and induce yourself, by using the Mirror exercise, (caduceus exercise) look at yourself between the third eye tell yourself mentally to go backward, stop, go forward, go backward, go forward, your arms are getting light.

4). Now look at the reflection of the light in the mirror, and observe it for atleast 30 seconds, just feeling your body.

5). Now look infront of you with open eyes and you will see the trace of light appear in the mirror.

6). Looking at the trace of light, ask your question.

7). Let the first answer that comes to you be your answer.

8). Keep asking your questions and let whatever appears appear.

9). When done, Close your eyes, put your hand on your belly.

10). Open your eyes sit down, interlock your fingers palms down and put your hands down a little below the navel with the palms down.

11). Search inside yourself and find some warm place.

12). When you find it imagine burning every image you saw and the energy going up along your spine.

13). When you are ready open your eyes.

Magnetism Of Objects

Any article of clothing can be magnetized and then if the person is susceptible when they put that article of clothing on they will fall into the mesmeric sleep, and heal. This is great when you are not available to work on the person directly.

To Do:

Just make passes with contact over the clothing and then hold it in your hands for a few minutes. You can make the effects last longer by keeping the clothes on you for a day or 2.

Magnetic Protection

You can also use magnetism to create protective amulets to stop a person from being magnetized by another. Generally to do this you want to have something that is real gold as this works the best. The magnetizer must magnetize with passes over and over putting in the protective intention. When he feels he is done. He may give the necklace or item back to the person and they must wear it at all times. This will prevent another person from being able to mesmerize them, including the person who magnetized the object. In order for the mesmer to mesmerize the person again the person must first remove the object.

Remember that the charge is not permanent and does wear off so it must be re-magnetized from time to time.

Final Thoughts

I hope this book, though small as it is, will guide you in healing those around you and give you the abilities to help heal yourself. Mesmerism has many uses and this book is just the beginning, but it is my sincere hope that it both gives you the tools to help others, and also opens your eyes and mind to the possibility of even more abilities with study and research. To get you started look into **Anton Mesmer, Count Alessandro di Cagliostro, Erminio di Pisa, Baron Du Potet, Louis Alphonse Cahagnet, and Armand-Marie-Jacques de Chastenet, the Marqués de Puységur.** These are all pioneers in mesmerism and should be a good start. They wrote books and you should find many interesting things within them.

Man was meant to be whole and healthy, he is one with the divine and always remember as we said in the beginning mesmerism is a gift of the divine. Use it well.